OCT 1 6

Praise for *Prevent, Survive, Thrive*

"Dr. West's book is a valuable addition to the current literature for those touched by breast cancer. He has dedicated his career to caring and healing women with breast cancer, which he reveals with knowledge and passion in this excellent book."

—John S. Link, MD, author of *The Breast Cancer Survival Manual: A Step-By-Step Guide for the Woman with Newly Diagnosed Breast Cancer*

"*Prevent, Survive, Thrive* continues Dr. John West's longstanding message of empowerment to those facing or in fear of breast cancer. This literary gift moves from prevention to survivorship to activism in sharing pearls of wisdom that transform us from victims to victors! This book is a wellspring of knowledge from a breast health leader who is a living legend in the fight against breast cancer. I am truly blessed to have witnessed John lead a breast health movement from his base in Orange County, California, to a national level."

—Marie M. La Fargue, MPH, four-time cancer survivor

"If you never want to hear the words, 'You have breast cancer,' this book is for you. You won't need a second opinion to decide whether to buy *Prevent, Survive, Thrive*. This book truly is, as it says on the cover, *Every Woman's Guide to Optimal Breast Care*. It helps you navigate confusing medical jargon and separates facts from the media buzz. There are plenty of books on facing the diagnosis of breast cancer, but this book, with its accurate straight-talk information, practical tips, and survivor stories filled with hope, helps you to prevent breast cancer. Every woman with breasts needs to read this book, and don't say this because it's funny. I say this because it's true."

—Pam Tallman, columnist and contributor to *Orange Coast Magazine*

"I wish I'd had this book at my fingertips years ago, but I am truly grateful for its publication at this time for the sake of my friends and family, as well as all women, both younger and older. Told in a blend of decades-rich expertise and personal case studies, this book provides a way to wrap your head around a woman's most dreaded health worry. *Prevent, Survive, Thrive: Every Woman's Guide to Optimal Breast Care* helps you sort through often conflicting reports and find your way to making better decisions."

—Allene Symons, author of *Aldous Huxley's Hands*

"Dr. West has shared his extensive experience in this uniquely comprehensive and easy-to-read treatise on all aspects of breast care for women of all ages (teens through seniors) and their loved ones, allowing them to be diligent in making decisions and their own choices regarding the ever-evolving questions of controversy and myth about breast cancer diagnostic alternatives and treatments. With the book's information on new technologies and multiple case histories, a patient can and should feel in charge of her own breast health plan in coordination with her chosen expert medical professionals."

**—Dr. Gary E. Liebl, LHD, chairman emeritus,
Chaminade University**

"My husband, Bill, and I as well as our family are very honored to have Dr. West's book *Prevent, Survive, Thrive* dedicated to our daughter Michelle, who lost her battle to breast cancer at the age of 26. A year after her death, we opened a Women's Breast Cancer Resource Center named Michelle's Place to offer resources and support to the women in the Temecula Valley area. It had been so difficult to find any when Michelle was going through treatment. We met Dr. West through our educational seminars because he had so many patients from our area that loved him! He is their rock star for sure! He shared our concern that more women needed to be their own best advocate and that knowledge is power. His book, *Prevent, Survive, Thrive*, meets these concerns and so many more! He writes so lay people can easily understand the many facets of breast cancer."

**—Bill and Marilyn Watson, founders of Michelle's Place,
a women's breast cancer research center**

Prevent
Survive
Thrive

Prevent
Survive
Thrive

EVERY WOMAN'S GUIDE TO
OPTIMAL BREAST CARE

Breast Care Surgeon

JOHN G. WEST, MD

with Maralys Wills

BENBELLA

BenBella Books, Inc.
Dallas, TX

BenBella Books, Inc.
10440 N. Central Expressway, Suite 800
Dallas, TX 75231
www.benbellabooks.com
Send feedback to feedback@benbellabooks.com

Printed in the United States of America
10 9 8 7 6 5 4 3 2 1

Library of Congress Cataloging-in-Publication Data

Names: West, John G. (John Gilbert), 1941- author. | Wills, Maralys, author.
Title: Prevent, survive, thrive : every woman's guide to optimal breast care
    / John G. West with Maralys Wills.
Description: Dallas, TX : BenBella Books, Inc., [2016] | Includes
    bibliographical references and index.
Identifiers: LCCN 2016025092 (print) | LCCN 2016029574 (ebook) | ISBN
    9781942952237 (hardback) | ISBN 9781942952244 (electronic)
Subjects: LCSH: Breast—Cancer—Prevention—Popular works. | Women—Health
    and hygiene—Popular works. | BISAC: HEALTH & FITNESS / Diseases / Cancer.
    | HEALTH & FITNESS / Women's Health. | MEDICAL / Diagnosis. | MEDICAL /
    Health Risk Assessment.
Classification: LCC RA645.C3 W47 2016 (print) | LCC RA645.C3 (ebook) | DDC
    616.99/449—dc23
LC record available at https://lccn.loc.gov/2016025092

Editing by Eryn Carlson and Leah Wilson
Copyediting by Elizabeth Degenhard
Text design by Publishers' Design and
    Production Services, Inc.
Text composition by PerfecType, Nashville, TN

Proofreading by Amy Zarkos and
    Laura Cherkas
Indexing by Debra Bowman Indexing Services
Cover design by Sarah Dombrowsky
Printed by Lake Book Manufacturing

Distributed by Perseus Distribution
www.perseusdistribution.com

To place orders through Perseus Distribution:
Tel: (800) 343-4499   Fax: (800) 351-5073
E-mail: orderentry@perseusbooks.com

This book is dedicated to the memory of Michelle Watson, who was twenty-three years old when she was diagnosed with metastatic breast cancer. Though she first noticed a breast lump at age twenty-one, her doctors told her she was too young for breast cancer.

The correct diagnosis was never considered until a bone scan indicated she had metastatic cancer. She died at age twenty-six.

Michelle's parents are on a mission to improve the quality of breast care in the United States. This book was written in an effort to help them accomplish their mission.

Acknowledgments

John:

The inspiration for writing this book came from my patients. Their stories have taught me more about medicine than all the textbooks I have read and the lectures I have attended.

The book could not have been written if it were not for the support from my wife, Jan West, RN. She gave me the encouragement to start the project and provided ongoing support until the last words were written.

I've had support from so many friends, family, and patients that it is not practical to mention them all, but a few deserve special acknowledgment.

Breast care has reached the level of complexity that it takes a team to ensure optimal care and the same was true for this book. My physician support team included Drs. June Chen (breast radiologist), Michael Schoen (pathologist), John Link (breast oncologist), and Nimmi Kapoor (surgical oncologist). Their patience and expertise are greatly appreciated.

Technical support was also essential. Special thanks to Steven A. Feig, MD (the mammography controversy); Joel Moskowitz, PhD (cell phones); Evrin Ruzic, MD (organ transplant); Tim Taylor, PhD (toxicology); Kimberly Banks, MS, CGC, MBA (genetics); and Jennifer Swisher, PA (genetics). It should be noted that I take full responsibility for how I interpreted the advice they provided.

A special thanks to my many friends who were so gracious with their time and talent. The short list includes: Gary Liebl, LHD, and

Helen Hess (legal) were of great help in clarifying technical details. Abra Negreti and Judy Herrick helped fine-tune the final draft. Tracy Frantz provided insightful comments on what it is like to have a young daughter with a cell phone–related breast cancer. Maralyn Watson was gracious in sharing details about her daughter, Michelle.

I was also fortunate to be assisted by the BenBella team, who were highly professional and a joy to work with. Special thanks to Leah Wilson and Eryn Carlson, who walked me through the progression of transforming my draft proposal into an intelligible book. The process was grueling, but they made it all worthwhile.

Finally, I would like to express my appreciation to Maralys Wills, who is a patient, a friend, and a gifted writer. It was clear from the start I needed help on this project. When Maralys agreed to come on board, I knew we had a winning team. Without her experience and expertise, this book would never have come to print.

Maralys:
As always, I'm indebted to my husband, Rob, who accepts—nay, maybe enjoys—a kind of bachelorhood while I'm writing a book. But he goes beyond acceptance: He takes me out often for dinners, and he's apt to say, "I'm fine down here, babe. Go back upstairs and work."

With thanks to my critique group, who read each chapter and offered much-needed advice: Allene, Pam, Barbara, and P.J., who understood perfectly what we were trying to do. But a special thanks to the two men, Erv and Terry, who were not appropriately equipped but were willing, nonetheless, to take the long view on the presentation.

Thanks, also, to numerous family and friends who listened patiently as I enumerated various little speed bumps in the project.

Contents

Why This Book Was Written

O F THE MANY STORIES from my forty-plus years of practice, one in particular stands out in memory: that of a young woman named Michelle Watson, who at twenty-one noticed a lump in her right breast.

Alerted by the nodule, Michelle saw the doctor in her student health clinic, who told her not to worry. He pointed out that she was the picture of health . . . and besides, she had no family history of breast cancer.

The lump continued to grow. Over the next two years she was seen by several other doctors, all of whom said her fears were unfounded, that she was too young for breast cancer.

At age twenty-three she experienced pain in her chest and back. The pain progressed, and finally a bone scan revealed what nobody had anticipated—Michelle had extensive metastatic disease. A subsequent biopsy of her breast lump, now grown to a considerable size, proved all those earlier medical assumptions wrong. Right from the beginning she'd harbored an invasive breast cancer.

She underwent aggressive chemotherapy, but her cancer recurred, and at age twenty-six she died of metastatic disease.

Michelle's death might very well have been preventable. Had she insisted on an ultrasound during her first office visit, her cancer could have been diagnosed while it was still potentially curable.

Michelle's story is an extreme case, but it sends an important message, one that is central to this book. When it comes to achieving optimal care, women must be prepared to take charge of their health—which includes knowing more about their breasts than some physicians.

In the past decade, remarkable progress has been made in improving the effectiveness of breast care. Ironically, this progress has led to a myriad of confusing and conflicting—and even misleading—recommendations about what women should do to ensure they are receiving optimal care. Such confusion often provokes diagnostic delays, resulting in the need for more aggressive treatments and lower odds of survival.

Although I've spent most of my career caring for women with breast issues, I started private practice with a focus on vascular and emergency surgery. In my first year, an event occurred that radically changed my life.

After an auto accident, an eight-year-old boy was brought to the emergency room of a local hospital. He was stable on admission, but in less than an hour he went into shock. He was rushed to the operating room but died before the surgeon could control the bleeding from his ruptured kidney.

I'd done my surgical training in San Francisco, where all serious trauma victims were transported to a single trauma center that had an in-house team of experts. Had this young boy been taken to a trauma center, he would most likely be alive today.

This needless loss of a young life prompted me to do a study comparing trauma deaths in Orange County, California, where trauma victims were transported to the nearest emergency room, to trauma deaths in San Francisco, where all serious trauma victims were taken to a trauma center. The study found that one-third of the total deaths in Orange County were judged to be preventable, but no preventable deaths were found in patients triaged to the trauma center.

This study inspired a worldwide focus on the importance of organizing civilian trauma care like the military MASH (mobile army surgical hospital) units during the Vietnam era. Orange County subsequently established a system of trauma care that became a model for the nation. A follow-up study proved the new system had solved the problem of preventable deaths in Orange County.

After ten years of promoting the concept of trauma centers, I experienced burnout: too many late-night surgeries and too little sleep. I was in urgent need of a change in lifestyle.

At the same time, a revolution was taking place in the diagnosis and treatment of breast cancer. Studies had proved radical mastectomies were rarely indicated, as similar rates of survival could be achieved with less aggressive surgery. Mammography was finding breast cancers years before lumps could be detected. Plastic surgeons were making major strides in breast reconstruction. Oncologists had new drugs that were more effective and less toxic.

Yet despite these advances, care was fragmented. Breast radiologists, breast surgeons, and breast oncologists were all in different offices and rarely had time to talk to each other. This was the opportunity I was looking for: Like trauma care, breast care needed organization.

I became obsessed with the concept of establishing a center that would address all aspects of care at one location. The basic team would include radiologists who specialized in imaging, together with surgeons and oncologists whose only focus would be breast care. The concept included a same-day model in which patients with new problems could be seen within a day of their call to our center.

We opened our first breast center in 1988, originally called Breast Care Center of Orange, and since then we have diagnosed and treated thousands of women with cancer and tens of thousands of patients with other breast issues.

It soon became obvious that the breast center concept was saving lives. Women who followed early detection guidelines were typically diagnosed with small, curable cancers—though the situation was much different for women who did not follow the guidelines.

The majority of advanced malignancies that we cared for occurred in women who had never had a mammogram or had neglected to have one for years. The conclusion was obvious: Aggressive screening worked. The challenge was to figure out how to get more women to participate in our early detection efforts.

My initial approach was to help establish a nonprofit organization (the Be Aware Foundation) in 2004 with the goal of inspiring women to follow early detection guidelines. We presented classes on breast self-examination and created a video to help women learn how to do self-exam with confidence. We also created a website where women could sign up for monthly reminders to do self-exam and a yearly reminder to get a mammogram and clinical exam. I wrote frequent articles, sent out with the monthly email reminders, dealing with the evolving controversies in breast care.

Despite my best efforts, the campaign to get more women to follow early detection guidelines was being thwarted by forces beyond my control. Our own government was promoting watered-down screening guidelines. Well-respected nonprofit organizations that in the past were proponents of early detection were issuing their own weakened recommendations.

The media was having a great time reporting all this conflicting advice. As a result, public confusion mounted. The net result was that fewer women were following early detection guidelines and diagnostic delays were on the upswing.

I became increasingly frustrated that women were receiving so many mixed messages. It was that ongoing frustration, plus the desire to set the record straight, that prompted me to write this book. To me it was obvious that something must be done to fight back against the "experts" who were the source of so much confusion. I wanted to inspire women to follow early detection guidelines and demand optimal breast care.

That said, I did not want to write something encyclopedic . . . and I had no interest in being "fair and balanced."

I wanted to compose a work that easily explains issues in the same manner I use in answering questions from my own patients. As I was wrestling with my approach, I had an appointment with a woman recently diagnosed with breast cancer. After I completed my lengthy explanation of treatment options, I was greeted by a long pause in which I could tell she was having problems processing our discussion.

She then looked me straight in the eye, and with a newfound confidence she said, *"Just tell me what you would do if I were your wife."*

The advice I gave her that day was the same I would offer members of my own family—mother, wife, or daughter.

And then I thought further: While it's relatively easy to advise my own patients, what about the millions of women who are desperate for information but don't know where to find it?

I hope that this book—written from the point of view of not just a breast care surgeon, but also a husband and father—will be a helpful resource for those women and their families.

THE PLAN BEHIND THE BOOK

For the convenience of our readers who wish to find breast care information quickly and easily, this book is organized in a way that makes it easy to get answers to a wide spectrum of breast care issues. To help bring these topics to life, most chapters are illustrated with one or more personal stories of women who have experienced the issues we describe.

We begin with specific issues that may arise, and recommendations for treatment, for women (and men) according to their age. Subsequent chapters address common breast problems, then uncommon but perilous breast problems. This is followed by a brief exploration of the various controversies in breast care as well as a brief discussion on prevention. Further chapters provide guidelines for women who are newly diagnosed, including when you may need a second opinion. Finally, we describe surgical options and offer a discussion of breast reconstruction, before concluding with the importance of hope when it comes to winning the battle against breast cancer.

CHAPTER ONE

The Controversies That Drive This Book

THE QUESTION of what constitutes optimal breast care—noted briefly in the Introduction—is not just an idle subject that is open for debate; it is now one of the most contentious issues in all of medicine.

Despite incredible progress everywhere in diagnosing and treating breast cancer, guidelines for optimal breast care today are brimming with contradictions and misleading statements. There is a growing trend to cut back on early detection efforts, based partly on flawed scientific studies, but also, regrettably, on cost. While it's true that medical costs are spiraling out of control, any procedural change that contributes to giving cancer a greater foothold will ultimately be more expensive for everyone.

Among the biggest controversies are the following:

Screening Mammography

Clearly the most outrageous controversy I've witnessed was promoted by the doctor who proclaimed on Fox News that mammograms can do more harm than good and stated that one in five cancers will disappear without treatment. The reasoning behind his fallacious statement and the proof of its nonsense will be demonstrated in chapters fifteen and sixteen.

Yet other controversies have made mammograms the subject of dangerous confusion. Traditionally, women have been told that they need to begin mammograms at age forty and continue yearly.

Now a government task force, the USPSTF (United States Preventive Services Task Force), offers new, reduced-mammogram guidelines that contradict reliable, proven standards (see chapter sixteen). The USPSTF recommends that mammogram screening start at age fifty, that it be repeated only every other year, and that it be discontinued after age seventy-four—even though none of the research has suggested that routine screening be discontinued at any age as long as a woman is in good health. None of the so-called "experts" on the USPSTF were physicians whose specialty was breast care.

Breast Density

For women whose mammograms show they have dense breasts, a second and different type of screening can detect tumors not seen on traditional mammograms. Yet, thanks to a mix of small additional cost and disbelief by so-called experts that this second screening is necessary, only a small fraction of the female population with dense breasts ever get the additional screening they need (see chapter fourteen).

Breast Self-Examination

Perhaps the least-expected controversy concerns two nonprofit organizations—the Susan G. Komen foundation and the American Cancer Society (ACS)—who concluded jointly that breast self-examination does not work, and therefore women no longer need to do self-exams (see chapter thirteen). Instead, they suggest women should be "self-aware" and report any change. How confusing can it get?

Genetic Testing

In 2013, Angelina Jolie went public with her announcement that she carried a high-risk gene mutation and had decided to have both breasts removed. At the time, the cost of genetic testing was in the range of $4,000. Now, only a few years later, any woman can be tested for $249—and she can apply online. Yet too few women are aware of the lowered cost or even that such knowledge might help guide their health care decisions.

Why So Many Mastectomies?

There is a growing trend for women who have been diagnosed with a malignancy to choose a mastectomy, even when they are ideal candidates for saving their breast. Oftentimes this decision is based on the assumption that mastectomy will provide better potential for survival—but this assumption is misguided. (See chapter twenty-four.)

Cell Phones and Breast Cancer

Among breast care physicians and radiologists working in my field, there is a growing perception that cell phones worn for long periods in direct contact with the breast are a possible cause of breast cancer. However, like early observations from long-gone doctors about the harmful effects of smoking, this suspicious relationship has been refuted by physicians whose areas of concentration are in other fields. In fact, all suggestions of a causal relationship between cell phones and breast cancer have been laughed at by a great many doctors. (See chapter seventeen.)

AS MORE AND MORE of these breast-care controversies surfaced, I began to think, *No wonder women are confused. How can I remain silent?* I've had too many years of experience to allow these many contradictions to go unanswered.

I am admittedly at one end of the spectrum on these ongoing con-flicts: My primary goal is to expand efforts to detect breast cancer at its earliest, most lifesaving stage. Although most experts would agree with me in principle, the advice some are giving women often gets in the way of this goal.

I hope the pages that follow give you the information you need to make your own decisions about how best to protect your health.

General Breast Care Guidelines by Age and Sex

CHAPTER TWO

For Children, Teens, and Women Under Forty

Just as "ONE SIZE FITS ALL" doesn't work in clothing, neither does it work in breast care. As you'll see in this section, different rules apply to different age groups—and what might be considered optimal care for one group can be detrimental to another.

Women in their thirties, for instance, whose breasts tend to be dense, are screened differently than their older sisters . . . and for them breast care deals primarily with the treatment of symptoms. Though we do address pain, infection, and nipple discharge, the most important issue is lumps.

While younger women are advised not to get routine screening mammograms, they are also, happily, less apt to acquire breast cancer. However, those who do find suspicious lumps are under more pressure to act quickly.

On the other hand, by age forty, women have crossed a line that divides "younger" from "older" women. While X-ray diagnosis is no longer a safety issue, the possibility of developing breast cancer is high enough to justify the expense and inconvenience of screening mammograms.

This section outlines what can be expected in women's breast history from newborns through the years until the woman turns forty. In each age group, a discussion of possible breast concerns is followed by recommended treatment options.

NEWBORNS

Breast Lumps

Breast lumps are common in newborns. They are almost always benign and related to maternal hormones encountered in the womb. In some cases, milk can be expressed from the nipple. The effect is short-lived and the breast soon returns to normal. Referral to the pediatrician is indicated if symptoms persist after several weeks. In the rare case in which the baby has a fever and the breast is red and swollen, the pediatrician should be contacted immediately.

PRE-TEENS

Breast Lumps

Pre-teen girls usually develop a button-like prominence directly below the nipple. At first, the lump may be evident on one side only. This is a common finding in young women entering puberty. The "lump" is referred to as a breast bud. Observation is all that is required. When we see this type of lump in our office we simply inform the parents to return in one to two months if they still have any questions or concerns. Surgical removal of the breast bud will result in the failure of breast development.

Lumps that aren't breast buds in pre-teens are unusual and require the attention of a physician. An ultrasound is the diagnostic procedure of choice for any persistent lump in this age group. An experienced surgeon, preferably a pediatric surgeon, should be involved in the decision-making process.

In select cases a needle biopsy should be performed to establish a diagnosis. Follow-up treatment will be based on the results of the needle biopsy.

Asymmetry

It is common for one breast to develop faster than the other. In most cases, reassurance is all that is required. An exam by the pediatrician is sufficient to reassure the patient and her family that all is well.

Breast Infections

Breast infections are rare in this young age group, and typically respond to antibiotics. Cases that are recurrent or unresponsive to therapy should be referred to a breast surgeon.

PUBERTY TO TWENTY

Breast Pain

Breast development and the onset of the menstrual cycle are indicators of early puberty. The pediatrician easily manages most issues of breast care in this age group. Issues such as cyclic breast pain are best handled with reassurance. In some cases, anti-inflammatories or caffeine restriction is advised (see chapter six).

Breast Lumps

Breast lumps are still unusual for this age group, but any such lump should be reported to the pediatrician. Although breast cancers are rare in teenagers, they do occur, and diagnostic delays must be avoided. Again, ultrasound is the diagnostic procedure of choice and mammograms are rarely indicated. A needle biopsy is usually needed to make the final diagnosis. Surgical removal should be considered only after an accurate diagnosis.

Breast Infections

Though infections are unusual in this age group, they are now being seen with increasing frequency as a result of nipple piercings. These infections usually respond to antibiotics. However, we've had cases in which the infection did not go away, requiring removal of the nipple ring. In some cases, the infection can lead to a disfiguring scarring of the nipple. Any sign of redness, pain, or swelling should be reported immediately and treated aggressively with antibiotics.

Radiation Exposure

It is well established that the developing breast is very sensitive to radiation exposure. Studies of women who, when they were teens, were treated for scoliosis (curvature of the spine) and had frequent chest X-rays to evaluate the progression of their disease show them to be at increased risk of developing a future breast cancer. X-rays cause direct damage to the DNA in the cells of the developing breast, an onslaught that sets the stage for future development of an early-onset breast cancer.

Now every effort is made to avoid X-ray exposure to the breasts of young women. When such treatment is required, the breasts are shielded with lead drapes. The dangers of radiation slowly diminish with the years, and by age thirty the risk is reduced to the point that it is safe to do a diagnostic mammogram when cancer is strongly suspected.

Young women who have had chest radiation for other malignancies are also at risk for early-onset cancer. The most common incidents are in girls who, during their teens or early twenties, receive chest wall radiation for the treatment of Hodgkin's disease.

Such women are often unaware of their risks and fail to follow early detection guidelines. Those who have been exposed to therapeutic radiation for Hodgkin's disease or other malignancies should be followed by experienced physicians, preferably in clinics that manage patients who are at increased risk of tumors. In addition to twice-yearly exams by an experienced physician, yearly MRI screening should start as early as age twenty-five. Yearly screening mammography should start as early as age thirty.

Radiation associated with cell phone exposure is an issue of recent controversy. See chapter seventeen to learn more about this debate.

WOMEN TWENTY TO THIRTY

Breast Lumps

Breast cancer is unusual in this age group. It does occur, however, and because of its rarity, diagnostic delays are common. The breasts in young women tend to be lumpy and tender, anyway, and most such women are not confident in doing breast self-examination.

A diagnostic ultrasound—the extreme value of which is described at length in chapter fourteen—is particularly accurate in defining the nature of a breast lump at any age. It works with sound waves, which are completely safe, as compared to X-rays employed by mammograms. It is also painless and inexpensive.

In most cases of concern about a potential breast lump, a normal ultrasound along with a negative breast exam is all that is needed. However, if symptoms persist, the patient should be referred to a surgeon with experience in caring for young women with breast problems.

Nipple Discharge

As will be discussed in chapter nine, nipple discharge that occurs on its own, without squeezing, requires medical attention, as it could be an early sign of cancer, except in the case of pregnant women or women who have just given birth.

OTHER BREAST PROBLEMS, such as pain and infection, are treated much the same in all age groups.

The key point to remember is that any new breast change that persists after a woman has completed her menstrual cycle should be reported to her physician. If her doctor is unresponsive to her concerns, she should seek a second opinion, preferably from a breast surgeon.

WOMEN THIRTY TO FORTY

Breast Lumps

Though breast lumps are common in women in their thirties, the good news is most prove to be benign. However, differentiating between benign and malignant can be challenging—generally because breasts in this age group, as with younger women, tend to be lumpy under normal circumstances.

Here, the menstrual cycle plays a role, adding both lumpiness and tenderness just before the onset of menstruation. That said, the best time to do a breast exam or evaluate a lump is five to ten days after the onset of the period.

And the best way to evaluate the seriousness of a nodule is with an ultrasound. If the diagnosis still remains sketchy, a diagnostic mammogram can be both helpful and safe.

This focused mammogram, covering a specific worrisome area, can be distinguished from a screening mammogram, which is done on women forty and over who have not experienced symptoms.

Breast Pain

Though breast pain is common in this age group, it's rarely associated with an underlying malignancy. Most such pain can be alleviated with over-the-counter anti-inflammatories, as well as caffeine restriction. Pain that is localized in one spot and increases in intensity over one or two menstrual cycles merits medical attention.

Breast Infections

Breast infections in this age group are typically associated with lactation, discussed in chapter four. Infections in non-lactating women

SCREENING MAMMOGRAMS FOR WOMEN UNDER FORTY

Compared to younger age groups, women in their thirties do have a somewhat higher occurrence of breast cancers. Since their breasts still tend to be dense, small malignancies don't show up well on mammograms.

For all these reasons, routine screening mammograms are not recommended, and a diagnostic ultrasound remains the first line of defense.

However, there are exceptions: Mammographic screening in this age group is restricted to women who have a first-degree relative (mother or sister) who was diagnosed with breast cancer under the age of fifty. Screening for those women should start ten years earlier than the age at which the relative was diagnosed. For example, if the mother was found to have a malignancy at age forty-five, the daughter would start yearly screening at age thirty-five.

In addition, very high-risk women, such as Angelina Jolie, who had multiple family members with breast and ovarian cancers and who tested positive for the BRCA gene mutation, require more aggressive screening. We follow these women twice yearly in our high-risk clinic, and we start yearly MRI screening at age twenty-five and yearly screening mammograms at age thirty.

Most of these women are also encouraged to consider risk assessment counseling, and in some cases, genetic testing (see chapter eighteen).

usually respond well to antibiotics. Those that don't, or that recur after initial treatment, should be seen by a breast care specialist.

OTHER SYMPTOMS in this age group, such as nipple discharge, are managed in much the same manner as with younger women.

WHAT I'D TELL MY DAUGHTER

- The vast majority of breast problems in this age group (birth to forty) will be associated with non-cancerous conditions.
- Still, breast changes merit attention. Persistent or progressive changes need a timely answer.
- When in doubt, get an opinion from a breast care specialist.

CHAPTER THREE

For Women Over Forty

THERE IS OBVIOUS OVERLAP when treating breast symptoms in the various age groups. For example, the care of symptomatic women in their thirties is nearly identical to what is offered for patients in their forties. To avoid repetition, we have simply summarized basic treatment in this and the previous chapter. A more detailed discussion of common breast problems is provided in Section II.

However, women in their forties should be aware of these concerns in particular:

Breast Lumps

Any new breast lump in a woman over forty merits concern. The older she is, the higher the probability of cancer. In menstruating women, breast lumpiness is common, but any nodule that persists after completion of a menstrual period requires medical attention. An ultrasound is often the only test needed to determine the nature of the lump. However, if doubt remains, a diagnostic mammogram is the next step. When findings on the mammogram or ultrasound are worrisome, a core needle biopsy (see page 48) will establish an accurate diagnosis.

If all diagnostic studies are negative, a further, two-month re-evaluation is still important, both to reassure the patient and to guard against a possible missed diagnosis of malignancy.

Abnormal Mammograms

The second most common breast problem in this age group is an abnormal screening mammogram. In most cases, additional imaging will eliminate concerns and the woman can return to routine yearly screening.

In the event of a positive finding, a core needle biopsy (see page 47) will provide an accurate diagnosis. If the biopsy is benign, the patient returns to regular screening. However, if the biopsy proves positive, the patient is referred to a breast surgeon.

Nipple Discharge

Nipple discharge is common in over-forty age groups, and squeezing the nipples is the primary cause. It is normal for breast ducts to contain fluid, and it is common for the breast, when squeezed, to produce a drop or more of yellow, green, or white fluid from the nipple. Although this discharge is not worrisome, women are advised *not* to squeeze their nipples.

However, discharge that occurs spontaneously requires medical attention—though in most cases the event is not related to a hidden breast cancer. Still, we are concerned when the fluid is either clear or bloody. If the discharge is suspicious enough to warrant a biopsy, it usually turns out to be benign, or associated with small, potentially curable breast cancers. For a more detailed discussion, see chapter nine.

Breast Pain

Breast pain is one of the most common symptoms that send women to a breast care center. While it is unusual for a breast cancer to cause pain, it can be the first indicator of an underlying malignancy. Pain that is centered in one specific area and becomes more intense in a matter of weeks merits the attention of a specialist. For further details, see chapter six.

Breast Infections

Breast infections are relatively common in nursing women, an issue covered in chapter four.

In non-lactating females such infections are rare but require immediate medical attention. With most patients, the inflammatory process responds to standard antibiotics. After treatment, an attempt should be made to determine the root cause. Infections that don't respond to antibiotics, or episodes that recur, should be referred to a breast care specialist.

MAMMOGRAMS

One of the biggest breakthroughs in the history of women's health care was the development of screening mammography. Initial studies in the United States and Sweden demonstrated a 30 percent or greater reduction in breast cancer mortality for women undergoing screening mammography. With improvements in technology and a better understanding of who is at risk, there is now an incredible opportunity for making even more dramatic improvement in the rate of survival of this number-one cancer killer of young women.

That said, age is one of the critical factors that increases a woman's chance of developing breast cancer. The older she gets, the greater her peril. By forty, vulnerability has reached the point where it's appropriate to start routine annual mammographic screening—and as always, the goal is to detect small cancers before they cause symptoms or even before they grow large enough to be felt.

Despite the well-established benefits of mammographic screening, we're seeing an increasingly strident disagreement over several issues: the best age to start, how often women should be tested, and the proper age to quit. This controversy will be explored in more detail in chapters fifteen and sixteen. It is first necessary to understand the basics of mammographic screening.

Screening vs. Diagnostic Mammogram

One of the first issues that needs clarification is the difference between a screening and a diagnostic mammogram. The screening mammogram is for women who are symptom free. They have no suspected breast lumps, no new patterns of breast pain, no nipple discharge, and basically no newly revealed breast symptoms. Diagnostic mammograms, on the other hand, are for women who have breast symptoms.

Women who are about to undergo their yearly screening exam should make certain they alert the technician or support staff about any recently discovered breast problems. Such symptoms will be reported to the radiologist (mammographer), who will then determine what additional procedures might be helpful to evaluate the new issues.

When to Start Screening

Despite all this recent controversy, there is a general consensus that starting mammographic screening at age forty saves lives. A government funded task force is now recommending women start mammographic screening at age fifty. However, this approach ignores an important group of women.

Approximately 20 percent—one out of five—cancers we see in our practice are in women *under* fifty. Patients with cancer who started mammographic screening at age forty tend to be diagnosed with small, treatable breast cancers, while most of the advanced cancers are found in patients who have never had a mammogram.

Self-proclaimed "experts" who advise that screening start at age fifty have two reasons: One is that most women in their forties have such dense breasts on mammographic imaging (see chapter fourteen) that it's hard to find small cancers . . . and, besides, "we all know" that fewer women in their forties develop breast cancer than women over fifty. The other is the much-touted concern about the issue of false positive biopsies. When the radiologist sees a worrisome spot on the mammogram, a needle biopsy is recommended. It is well-known that many of these biopsies will prove to be benign. The chance of a false positive is higher for younger women, in large part because many of these women are receiving their first mammogram and there are no previous images to check. When previous films are available for comparison, the number of false positive biopsies drop.

As the critics of early screening point out, a great deal of anxiety occurs when a woman is told she needs a breast biopsy. They conclude that the anxiety associated with a false positive biopsy is just one more reason why starting screening at age forty is not justified.

The critics, however, are not fair and balanced. They manage to overlook the downside—the anxiety associated with a delayed diagnosis. In my experience, most women are willing to take the chance of a false positive when it's associated with a potential for detecting a breast cancer at an earlier stage—that interval when treatment is less aggressive and the probability of survival is improved. As one of my patients noted, "Both ways it's good news: Either my doctor caught a malignancy early, while it's easily treatable, or I learn I don't have cancer."

My advice to patients: Start mammographic screening at age forty and do it yearly. This advice applies to women at normal risk for breast cancer. Those with strong family histories or others who have been exposed to radiation at a young age are followed more aggressively, which may include yearly clinical exams starting at age twenty-one, yearly MRIs starting at age twenty-five, and yearly mammograms starting at age thirty.

BI-RADS CLASSIFICATION

The American College of Radiology established a standardized reporting system called BI-RADS (or Breast Imaging Reporting and Data System) that is used by all mammography centers in the USA—a major advance, as before we had such a system screening reports were often difficult to interpret. All mammogram reports are given a final BI-RADS score ranging from zero to six.

- A category 0 report means additional imaging is required.

- Categories 1 and 2 indicate a completely normal exam. A category 2 score means something is seen on the mammogram, like a cyst, but because it is inconsequential, the exam is still considered to be normal. For both categories, a one-year follow-up is recommended.

- Category 3 indicates the presence of something that is probably benign. A six-month follow-up is indicated.

- Categories 4 and 5 indicate a cancer is suspected (more so in 5 than in 4) and a biopsy is mandatory.

- Category 6 means the diagnosis of breast cancer has been made and further treatment is required.

How Often to Do Screening

There is also ongoing controversy about how often to do mammographic screening. Some guidelines suggest every other year is sufficient. I am not convinced and will not be until there is more data to prove that this is just as safe as yearly.

When to Stop Screening

Limited data indicates that screening beyond age seventy-four saves lives. The explanation for ever selecting this particular age as an endpoint is that previous studies arbitrarily stopped with women older than seventy-four. Despite the lack of proof, I recommend that yearly screening continue as long as a woman remains in good health.

Tips for Women Undergoing Screening

The most common complaint about screening mammography is the pain that occurs when the breast is compressed. Although many women breeze through the process, there are others who dread the anticipated discomfort. A few steps can be taken to reduce apprehension.

- Menstruating women should schedule their mammogram five to ten days after the onset of their period, when the breasts are least tender.
- Menopausal women who are on hormone replacement should consider stopping their hormones one week prior to the exam.
- All women who are concerned about discomfort should consider taking ibuprofen or their favorite anti-inflammatory an hour before the examination.
- If you had a bad experience with your previous mammogram, tell the person setting up the equipment. In some cases, an experienced technician can make adjustments that will improve the experience.

With this exam, two other issues become important. The first is underarm deodorant, which should be avoided the day of the procedure (and all traces of prior deodorant should be washed off). Particles in the product, such as aluminum, can cause confusion and may lead to needless additional views. The second issue is the need for convenient clothing; women should wear a two-piece outfit with an easily removable top.

New Advances in Screening

Critics eagerly point out that screening mammograms fail to visualize many breast cancers, and, unfortunately, they are correct. One of the most frustrating aspects of my practice occurs when one of my patients, who for years has followed all of the early detection guidelines, is diagnosed with a late-stage breast cancer (see chapter ten). Fortunately, this situation is unusual.

The good news is that recent technology is coming to the rescue. One of the major advances in detecting cancers missed on mammographic screening is adding additional screening for the approximately 50 percent of patients who, on mammograms, are found to have dense breasts (see chapter fourteen).

Studies have demonstrated that the number of small cancers detected in women with dense breasts almost doubles when ultrasound is added.

A second fallback is the breast MRI, which is even more effective than ultrasound in detecting small cancers missed on mammograms. Because of the cost and inconvenience, we limit screening MRIs to women who are at very high risk for developing cancer, such as Angelina Jolie.

A third advance is tomosynthesis, or 3-D mammography. The 3-D mammogram is just what it states. Rather than the standard 2-D image of the breast, multiple images are taken. The images are fed into a computer and a three-dimensional image is provided. One recent study concluded that 3-D detected 27 percent more cancers than did screening with 2-D mammograms. In addition, there was a 15 percent reduction in need to call women back for additional views.

My Advice on Mammograms

Although some experts might conclude that my approach to screening is overly cautious, I am convinced it will save lives and lead to less aggressive treatment. In the long run, I believe it will prove to be cost-effective, considering the rapid increase in the expense of chemotherapy drugs.

I do agree with critics that women should be given an informed choice. The reality is that most primary care physicians, who are likeliest to order screening studies, do not have time to provide the information necessary for fully informed consent.

Although our primary goal in detecting cancers in women forty and over is to diagnose them before symptoms occur, it is not always possible. This is especially true in the underserved population, not because mammograms don't work in this population, but because this population is less likely to participate in screening.

Knowing what to do about breast problems as they arise often means the difference between a potentially curable cancer and one in which the prognosis is poor. The answer to this problem is quite simple: Educate yourself. Just reading this book will provide you with more information than you will ever get from the vast majority of physicians.

WHAT I'D TELL MY DAUGHTER

- Start yearly mammograms at age forty (or earlier if high risk; see Appendix I).

- Start monthly self-exams at age twenty-one, and see your physician if you detect a new lump or other changes.

- Report spontaneous nipple discharge to your physician, but do not squeeze your breast looking for discharge.

- Breast pain is common so don't worry unless it is in one spot and increasing in intensity.

🌱

CHAPTER FOUR

For Women of Childbearing Age: Birth Control, Pregnancy, and Lactation

FINDING SMALL BREAST CANCERS during pregnancy and lactation is a huge challenge, mainly because significant changes take place in the size, shape, and texture of the breasts while women are pregnant or nursing. As a result, the diagnosis of breast cancer is often delayed, and delays can be associated with adverse consequences.

Since the problems of early detection during pregnancy are different from those of lactation, it is best to consider the two issues separately. However, this section covers a number of issues besides cancer. Amid lingering but mostly unfounded concern about birth control pills and breast cancer, we also discuss the surprising number of options for birth control that women now have available to them.

BIRTH CONTROL

The "pill" first became available to the public in 1960 and proved to be an immediate success. Despite ongoing controversies, its popularity has only increased with time. Millions of young American women are now on this medication and with good reason. Not only is the pill effective in protecting against an unwanted pregnancy, it also has other desirable benefits, including the reduction of mood swings, the limiting of heavy menstrual flow, the improvement of acne, and a lowering of the risk of developing ovarian cancer.

Although this form of birth control has proven to be safe and effective for the majority of women, it does have some limitations, and it is important that young women be aware of them. One significant concern is that the pill is not 100-percent effective. It is estimated that one in 100 women who take it will nevertheless become pregnant. The primary explanation for failure in some women is simple: Usually it's because they forget to take it on a daily basis.

Another worry is that the pill may influence a woman's risk of developing breast cancer. The standard combination tablet contains two hormones: estrogen and progesterone. Both are synthetic, or manmade, hormones, designed to match the two naturally occurring hormones in a woman's body. The first BCPs (birth control pills), which were introduced in the 1960s, contained high levels of estrogen. It was subsequently shown that high-estrogen medications were associated with an increased risk of breast cancers. Today's BCPs contain a much lower dose of estrogen—but even with these diminished doses, concerns linger about the pill's safety.

Recent studies have clearly demonstrated that, for the vast majority of healthy young women, these fears are unfounded. The modern combination pill has become the first choice in birth control for most young women up to the age of thirty-five.

However, some users should strongly consider other options. Certainly, if you have either a personal history or a strong family history of breast cancer, an estrogen-containing BCP should be avoided. For example, if your grandmother was diagnosed with breast cancer in her eighties, the risk is inconsequential. But if your mother or sister was diagnosed before the age of fifty, alternative methods of birth control need to be considered.

Women who are concerned about their personal risk should discuss other types of birth control with a doctor, or go to a family planning clinic to get additional, specific information. It is also worth noting that women sometimes overestimate their personal risk, so expert advice on this subject is valuable in making an informed choice.

Women with strong family histories of breast cancer should be evaluated in a high-risk clinic . . . and should also be counseled on the many options of non-hormonal approaches to birth control (such as IUDs, diaphragms, and spermicidal gels).

Other health care issues should be taken into account when deciding on the best form of birth control for a specific woman. Those with clotting problems, such as a history of blood clots in the veins of the leg, should avoid the combination pill. The same is true of women with a history of heart disease, such as high blood pressure or a stroke.

Age is another important consideration. Since the possibility of a malignancy increases with age, I generally recommend that women over thirty-five consider alternatives to the standard pill. In addition, health risks for taking the combination pill are further increased in females who smoke or are overweight.

Fortunately, there are safe alternatives to the standard combination pill. The "mini-pill" is the method of choice for most high-risk women. Besides containing no estrogen, it offers only a synthetic form of progesterone. The mini-pill is extremely effective when taken daily and avoids many of the potential side effects of the combination. This medication has become the preferred birth control choice for women over thirty-five.

The mini-pill is also ideal for women who are at risk of breast cancer because of a strong family history, or who previously had a high-risk biopsy. The same can be said for women with a history of clotting or heart issues. Finally, the mini-pill is the right choice for breast-feeding mothers, since it does not reduce the flow of breast milk as does the combination pill.

Of course, there are other practical reasons for not taking either. For the medication to work, it must be taken on a daily basis—ideally, at the same time each day. If you are concerned about your potential for missing a dose, other alternatives, such as intrauterine devices (IUDs) and contraceptive implants may be the practical answer.

A second limitation is that none of these pills protect against sexually transmitted diseases (STDs). Women who want protection from that possibility should insist their partner wear a condom.

At present, there is incredible competition for creating the ideal pill. As a result, a bewildering list of choices from different manufacturers are available for both the combination and the mini-pill. Although this multitude of possibilities may seem confusing at first, there are benefits to having so many options. If the first pill you select is not well tolerated, there are many alternatives.

One of these choices will almost certainly prove to be the correct one for you.

PREGNANCY

Baseline Mammogram

One matter of importance to women in their mid-thirties who are considering future pregnancies is deciding when to obtain a baseline mammogram. Since breast cancers are more difficult to detect during pregnancy, it is common sense that patient and doctor would want to know in advance if the patient is harboring a small cancer that cannot be detected on physical exam.

A PRE-PREGNANCY EXAM THAT SAVED A LIFE

The Giuliana Rancic story was an eye opener for me. Rancic, a television personality and anchor for E! News, has been very public about her personal problems with infertility. She explained to viewers that she had failed to get pregnant on two attempts at in-vitro fertilization (IVF). She subsequently announced that she had found a world-class expert on IVF and was going to give it one more try.

Even though she was only thirty-six at the time, Rancic's infertility specialist advised her to have a baseline mammogram before beginning IVF. Despite having no breast symptoms and no family history of cancer, she nevertheless complied with the doctor's order. All her fans know the rest of the story: A small cancer was detected. She cancelled her IVF, and her cancer was successfully treated. Subsequently, Rancic used a surrogate, and she is now the proud parent of a little boy named Edward Duke.

Had she not gotten the mammogram and instead proceeded with IVF, the story would not have had such a happy ending.

I now think it is appropriate to recommend a baseline mammogram for women in their mid-thirties or older who are thinking about getting pregnant. Women with dense breasts should also consider a screening ultrasound. In addition, those with a strong family history of breast or ovarian cancer should opt for a baseline MRI.

Detecting Breast Issues During Pregnancy

Breast cancers and other issues can be detected early in their evolution if pregnant women follow a short list of guidelines. Having confidence in what the normal breast feels like prior to the onset of pregnancy is the first step.

In general, as we've noted in other chapters, we advise non-pregnant women to do monthly self-exams five to ten days after the onset of their menstrual period, since this is the time when breasts are least lumpy. Learning what your normal breast feels like should be started months, if not years, before becoming pregnant. (Guidelines for doing breast self-exams with confidence are outlined in chapter thirteen.)

Just as a non-pregnant woman can learn the pattern of her normal breasts, it is also possible for a pregnant woman to have a clear mental image of evolving, normal changes as her pregnancy progresses.

One approach for a woman to keep track of changes is to review the breast exam with her caregiver at each prenatal checkup. This self-exam should be repeated on the same night as the office exam.

The breasts should also be examined between well-woman check-ups. It is normal to see changes as the pregnancy follows its usual course. As long as the changes seem symmetrical on both sides, it is reasonable to assume all is well. If, during the self-exam, one area seems to stand out from the rest, it should be rechecked daily for a few days.

If the area of concern persists, an appointment should be made to review these findings with a medical provider. In most cases, the woman will be reassured that the questionable area can be safely observed. Still, it's important to make a one-month follow-up appointment. This short interval is vital, because breast cancers can grow rapidly during pregnancy.

If, on the first visit, the caregiver agrees there is an area requiring further evaluation, the next logical step would be a diagnostic ultrasound. If the ultrasound appears abnormal, a referral should be made to a breast surgeon or a breast imager with expertise in dealing with complex breast problems.

For the majority of women, however, that one-month return office visit would be the next step. If the patient is still concerned about a particular area, again a directed ultrasound should be ordered, even if the physical exam seems normal to the clinician. Assuming the diagnostic ultrasound is negative, the patient can then return monthly for at least two more visits.

On the other hand, if symptoms persist and the exam and ultrasound remain negative, the next step is a diagnostic mammogram. Women can be reassured that the mammogram is perfectly safe as long as the abdomen is properly shielded with a lead blanket.

When the doctor notes a problem area on either the ultrasound or mammogram, tissue sampling is suggested, which is typically done with a large bore needle to get an adequate sample. Open surgical biopsy is rarely indicated.

Lactating Adenomas

Most breast biopsies done during pregnancy turn out to be benign. One example of a common benign solid lump is called a lactating adenoma. These lumps are actually more common in pregnancy than during lactation, thus the name is misleading.

Like most benign lumps that occur during this event, lactating adenomas can be safely observed once a needle biopsy has established the diagnosis. However, lactating adenomas may rapidly enlarge, and careful follow-up by an experienced surgeon is indicated. In some cases, rapidly growing benign solid lumps require removal, which is relatively safe if done during the second or third trimesters.

Breast Cancer Treatment During Pregnancy

In the rare case in which the core biopsy does reveal a breast cancer, the patient should be referred to a team of physicians and support personnel who are experienced in meeting the complex needs of a pregnant woman with breast cancer. A comprehensive treatment plan must take multiple factors into consideration, including the health of the mother and her unborn child. Issues regarding the timing of surgery and chemotherapy must be individualized to the patient's personal needs, based on the stage and aggressiveness of the cancer, as well as to the time period of the pregnancy.

It should be noted that both surgery and chemotherapy are considered safe for the mother and her unborn child after completion of the first trimester. Breast irradiation, however, is not safe.

BREAST ISSUES DURING LACTATION

Soon after delivery, the breasts become engorged with milk. They are swollen, lumpy, and seemingly impossible to examine with confidence. Fortunately, breast cancers are rare in lactating women. However, they do occur, and diagnostic delays are common.

During the first few weeks of lactation, the breasts are so engorged that it is impractical to attempt self-examination. However, over time the breast exam is more easily performed. The best time to do it is after nursing or pumping.

In my own practice I am often surprised by how easy it is to do a clinical exam of a woman who has "emptied" her breasts within the hour of her office visit. This observation leads me to conclude that once the early changes associated with the onset of lactation are resolved, breast self-exam is feasible, and is still the most effective method a woman has to protect herself against a delay in breast cancer diagnosis.

While breast problems are common during lactation, the vast majority are not related to cancer. One of the most frequently seen issues is a plugged milk duct, which can be relieved by applying warm compresses or breastfeeding, or with massage. Sometimes redness and pain develop, a condition called mastitis, in which case antibiotics are necessary.

For women in whom the inflammation does not resolve in a few days or seems to get worse under treatment, referral to a breast surgeon should be considered. Although inflammatory breast cancer (see chapter eleven) is rare, it should be considered in cases in which an inflammation does not respond to standard treatment.

Benign breast lumps that occur during lactation are of two basic types: cystic and solid. "Milk cysts" are those most commonly seen in my practice. They are easy to diagnose on ultrasound, and usually they will go away on their own. But if they are painful or of concern to the patient, they can be easily aspirated in the office under local anesthesia.

Solid breast lumps are also common during lactation. Ultrasound is the first step in evaluating new irregularities in nursing mothers. Solid lumps are easily distinguished from cystic lumps. Benign lumps (non-cancerous) are generally easy to distinguish from those that are suspicious.

Benign lumps are typically smooth and round, and for these I simply aspirate the lump with a fine needle and send the cells to the pathologist. If the review confirms that the cells are benign, I can easily monitor the patient's progress in my office. If, on physical exam or ultrasound, the mass in question is hard and irregular, I typically go straight to a core needle biopsy.

That said, open surgical biopsy should be avoided whenever possible. An open biopsy during lactation is fraught with problems because of dilated milk ducts and increased blood supply to the lactating breasts.

In rare cases, a breast cancer will be diagnosed during lactation. Just as with pregnancy, a team approach is essential for optimal outcomes. A nursing woman on chemo will need to stop breastfeeding, but can safely continue while on radiation as long as she uses only the non-radiated breast.

WHAT I'D TELL MY DAUGHTER

- The combination pill is an excellent choice for most women, but women should be aware of their personal risks and discuss other options with their physician.

- Continue to do monthly self-exam during pregnancy and lactation and report any persistent major changes to your physician.

CHAPTER FIVE

For Men

Yes, men can and do have breast problems. As with women, the vast majority are not related to cancer. It has been estimated that a young man has a better chance of winning the lottery than of being diagnosed with breast cancer . . . but surprisingly, it is possible.

The same can't be said for testicular cancer, the most common malignancy in males between the ages of fourteen and forty. So why mention testicular cancer in a chapter on breast issues in men? The reason is simple: A breast lump can be the first sign of a hidden testicular cancer.

A great deal of progress has been made in treating testicular cancer, but to maximize the potential for cure, it is still important to detect the malignancy at its earliest stage. Also, delays in diagnosis often result in the need for more aggressive treatment, which may include both chemo and radiation therapy.

In addition to the possibility of testicular cancer in young men, there is a chance of breast cancer in older men. As with women, age is a significant predictor of the types of breast problems males are likely to experience. Therefore, in discussing issues on the masculine side, it is logical to divide them into three age categories, recognizing there is a fair amount of overlap between the age groups.

NEWBORNS TO PUBERTY

It is common for newborn babies of both sexes to have enlarged breasts, and some will have lumps below their nipples. This is a self-limiting condition, and no treatment is required. In most cases, the enlargement will go away in a matter of weeks.

In the years between birth and the onset of puberty, breast problems are rare for both sexes. Still, breast lumps and breast infections can occur, and any changes should be reported to a pediatrician.

Puberty is when breast problems become more common in boys. Enlargement on one or both sides is often associated with pain, tenderness, and a distinct mass. A breast lump in this age group is referred to as gynecomastia, which roughly translates as "breasts like those of a woman."

The term gynecomastia is actually well chosen, because it implies a hormonal origin to the problem, which in fact is the case. The term is reassuring, since it avoids any reference to breast cancer, which is extraordinarily rare in this age group. A careful history and clinical exam of the breast is all it takes to make the diagnosis. In most cases, reassurance and observation are sufficient. Though the risk of missing a breast cancer in this age group is extraordinarily low, I still advise parents to have the child return if there is any progression of symptoms, such as an increase in size or onset of pain or tenderness. When gynecomastia lasts longer than two years, the chances of the breasts returning to normal are greatly reduced. We encourage boys with persistent small lumps to wait them out since, over the next few years, many of these lumps will slowly go away.

Larger lumps are more problematic. Often these protrusions are so obvious they are visible even when the boy is wearing a T-shirt. The embarrassment can be devastating to young boys, who are often already self-conscious about their body image.

With boys who have a large lump or whose entire breast is enlarged because of an excess of fatty tissue, it is more difficult to obtain a satisfactory cosmetic result. In these unusual cases, referral to a plastic surgeon may be indicated.

Although there are reports of gynecomastia cases responding to hormone-blocking medications, I have no personal experience with this approach. If the family has an interest in trying a medical approach, I would recommend consultation with an endocrinologist.

MEN FOURTEEN TO FORTY

When I see a young male with a breast lump in this age group, the first thing that comes to mind is the possibility of an associated testicular cancer. Missing such a cancer in a young man can be just as dangerous as missing the diagnosis of a breast cancer in a young woman.

Thus, every breast lump in this age group needs special attention, even though the chances of it being the first sign of hidden testicular cancer are small. The key to avoiding a delayed diagnosis is for the treating physician to consider testicular cancer as a possibility. Specific questions should be asked about any history of testicular symptoms, such as swelling, tenderness, pain, lumps, or any other oddity the patient can remember. An examination of the testicles should also be done. If there is even the slightest possibility of an abnormal finding on clinical exam, a testicular ultrasound should be ordered.

It is important to keep in mind that the testicular exam can be completely normal and still harbor a "hidden" cancer. These "occult" testicular malignancies are often first detected by blood-test screening in young men with breast enlargement.

I routinely order the following blood tests for young men with breast lumps:

- AFP (alpha-fetoprotein)
- Beta hCG (human chorionic gonadotropin)
- LDH (lactate dehydrogenase)

If any of the three tests are elevated, I refer the patient to a urologist. I will not schedule surgical removal of a breast lump in a young male until the blood tests come back as normal and the rest of the workup has been negative.

In my experience it is rare to find hidden testicular cancers in this group of patients. That being said, I have a vivid memory of one young man who died of metastatic testicular cancer. His prognosis would have been much more favorable if his condition had been diagnosed two years earlier when he presented with a breast lump.

From what I've seen, breast lumps in the fourteen-to-forty age group are frequently caused by medications, the most common being body-building steroids. Often these muscle-enhancing hormones are not clearly labeled on the products. As a result, many of the young men who come to me with a breast lump are not aware that the product they've been taking contains steroids or steroid-like compounds.

Stopping the use of steroids is helpful in some cases, but often the breast lump persists, even when all medications are eliminated.

Another common cause of male breast enlargement in this age group is marijuana. Most of my patients deny smoking it, and I don't push the issue. But I suspect more are using cannabis than are willing to admit it.

In this age group, there is also a long list of medications, noted in the chart below, that are associated with male breast enlargement. In some cases, stopping or switching medication helps, but again the results are unpredictable.

DRUGS THAT CAUSE GYNECOMASTIA

Category	Drugs
Hormone	Anabolic steroids, estrogen, androgen, growth hormone
Recreational Drugs	Marijuana, amphetamines, heroin
Anti-Ulcer Drugs	Cimetidine, Omeprazole, Ranitidine
CNS-Acting Drugs	Tricyclic antidepressants
Heart Medications	Digoxin, calcium channel blockers

As with adolescent males with breast lumps, men in this age group who experience a persistent lump have the choice of living with it or having it surgically removed. From my experience, the young men who choose surgical removal almost always have a favorable cosmetic result.

MEN FORTY AND OLDER

When I see a man in his forties or older with a new lump, I know the odds are high that it will not be cancer. Again, most of these lumps are caused by medications. The most common prescriptions associated with breast enlargement are those used to treat heart disease, prostate cancer, indigestion, and depression. But the list doesn't end there. It seems as though every commonly prescribed drug will list gynecomastia as a possible side effect. A predominance of men over forty are on at least one of these medications, and with age the list grows.

For the most part, my job is to make certain a breast cancer is not the cause of the lump. It is usually easy to determine. Benign breast enlargement in older men feels like a smooth, hard disc of tissue, whereas cancers are hard and irregular to the touch, and often associated with dimpling in the skin or nipple.

I recommend a mammogram for all men over forty who find lumps. I also include the same blood tests for testicular screening for men in their forties and fifties as I do for younger men.

The mammogram is highly accurate in making the diagnosis of gynecomastia. In the past, I typically did a core needle biopsy to confirm the diagnosis. I have become so confident about the accuracy of the imaging workup that I now do core biopsy only in select cases. All patients with this condition are encouraged to return as needed if they have questions, or if the lump continues to grow. I routinely suggest a six-month follow-up exam.

Imaging is also accurate in identifying changes in the breast that require some form of tissue sampling to rule out male breast cancer.

With these men I do an immediate core needle biopsy. Surgical removal is seldom needed for an accurate diagnosis.

In rare cases, the findings on the core biopsy are at odds with the findings on imaging, which means surgical removal is indicated.

Once a diagnosis of breast cancer is made, we discuss treatment options. Most older males choose mastectomy, but in select cases lumpectomy plus radiation is a reasonable alternative.

All males with invasive breast cancer should see an oncologist. These men should also get risk assessment and, in most cases, gene testing to determine if they carry a gene mutation.

One of the great problems in caring for males with breast lumps is that guys often are oblivious to changes in that area of their bodies. As a result, it is common for them to appear with large lumps that are distorting the shape of the breast and should be obvious to even a casual observer.

When I ask these fellows how long they have been aware of changes, they typically say they just noticed them. Yet the reality is they've probably been going on for a year or longer. Men just don't think about breast exams.

They seem blissfully unaware of the issue of male breast cancer. I am not recommending that men do routine monthly breast self-exams, but I believe men should at least make the effort to know what their normal breasts are like, and to become more proactive in reporting changes.

WHAT I'D TELL MY DAUGHTER

- Most lumps in teens and younger can be safely observed.
- Surgery is rarely indicated for gynecomastia.
- Tests for testicular cancer should be performed for new breast lumps in males ages fifteen to forty.
- New lumps in males forty and over should be evaluated for the possibility of breast cancer.

SECTION II

Common Breast Problems

CHAPTER SIX

Breast Pain

It's breast pain that most often brings patients to our clinic. Although the majority of such women will not have cancer, it is still essential for the physician to keep in mind that pain *can* be an early cancer symptom—and it's his or her responsibility to identify the rare patient whose pain is triggered by a hidden malignancy.

Breast soreness is most common in young women. It typically starts several days before the onset of menstruation and gets worse until the beginning of the period. That discomfort is generally associated with rising hormone levels, whereas the onset of the period is followed by a reduction in the intensity of the pain.

We refer to this pattern of pain as cyclic breast pain and it is considered normal. However, pain that occurs independent of the menstrual cycle is referred to as noncyclic breast pain and often requires medical attention.

A careful history is our starting point. I usually begin with the statement, "Describe the nature of your pain." I then become more specific: "How long have you had it? Is it stable or getting worse? Is it intermittent or continuous?"

A combination of symptoms raises my concern about the possibility of a developing breast cancer. The first clue is when the woman is precise about the location of concern. If the patient then informs me that the discomfort has been getting progressively worse over the past several weeks, I assume the pain is due to breast cancer until proven otherwise.

However, most women with discomfort have difficulty pointing to an area of maximum concern. Not only does its location seem vague, but the history is often difficult for the patient to describe. The big clue that the pain is not of malignant origin is when the pain does not increase in severity over a period of several weeks.

After taking a history, the next step is the physical exam. I ask the patient to point to the sensitive area before I start. Usually she finds it difficult to locate the exact area. With vague area of distribution, I am reassured the pain is not likely to be of malignant origin.

In most cases, the exam will be negative, but occasionally a lump will be noted of which the woman was not aware. Ultrasound will readily differentiate between cystic and solid masses. As stated earlier, we usually aspirate cysts. Solid masses require a more extensive evaluation, and some will require a core needle biopsy to make an accurate diagnosis. Fortunately, most will prove to be benign.

Assuming the physical examination is negative, I prefer to do an ultrasound directed to the areas of maximum soreness, which in most cases is normal. I have the patient look at the ultrasound image of the area and then study other areas of the breast that are pain free. It is reassuring for her to see that the area of worry looks exactly like the other normal areas in her breast.

For women in their mid-thirties and older, I either do a baseline mammogram or repeat the diagnostic mammogram if it has been more than six months. If all is normal, I recommend she return two, four, and six months following her first visit. I advise menstruating women to schedule the appointment five to ten days after the onset of their period. In most cases the pain is either gone or the pattern of discomfort remains stable and the patient can return to routine screening.

There is a small but important group of patients with breast pain who do not fit into this neat little pattern. In these rare instances, though both the physical exam and imaging may be normal, the pain progresses over time.

The next step, then, is to order a breast MRI. For practical purposes, a normal MRI essentially rules out the possibility of a hidden cancer as the cause of pain.

OTHER CAUSES OF BREAST PAIN

With some women, the cause of breast pain is not due to changes in the breast but is caused by structures or organs near the breast.

Discomfort can arise from the bones, muscles, and tendons of the chest wall, the shoulder joint, or the cervical spine. Soreness can also be caused by medical conditions, such as esophageal reflux or coronary artery disease.

In those few instances where the breast evaluation is negative and the pain persists, consideration should be given to seeing other specialists, such as an orthopedist or an internist. We have also seen benefits in referral to a pain center where nerve blocks or steroid injections are effective in relieving pain in the area of the breast. In other situations, acupuncture had significant benefits.

TREATMENT OF BREAST PAIN

Once we have established that the pain is not due to a definable problem within the breast, or to structures or organs near it, the treatment is designed to reduce the patient's symptoms. Women with cyclic breast pain are advised to take acetaminophen or their favorite anti-inflammatory, such as ibuprofen.

Women on birth control should think about switching to another brand of pill or even to another method, such as IUDs. Menopausal women on hormone replacement therapy might consider reducing the dose of their hormones.

Caffeine restriction is generally recommended, but studies to prove the value of this approach have been inconclusive. In my experience, women who are consuming four to five cups of coffee per day get relief when they minimize their caffeine intake. The benefit is typically less apparent in women who drink one or two cups a day.

The studies on vitamin E and evening primrose oil have also been inconclusive, but I still recommend them. Both are inexpensive and well tolerated, and many patients seem to benefit from taking them. It's a bit like taking chicken soup for a cold. It can't hurt, and with many patients it helps.

The one medication proven to be effective is danazol. Studies have demonstrated that this drug can reduce breast pain in about 70 percent of patients. The problem with danazol is its side effects, which include abnormal growth of body hair and lowering of the voice. In my experience, women who read the package insert rarely go on to take the medication. It is a reasonable, but temporary, choice for women with major breast pain that is unresponsive to other treatments.

Occasionally, one simple solution to relieve pain is to find a good-fitting bra. I remember one patient, Judy, who bought a twelve-dollar bra at Target. To her surprise, it was a "perfect fit" and was very effective in minimizing her discomfort. She even wore it at night. For some women, just finding the right bra seems to be all it takes.

Surgery for pain alone is rarely an option. However, I know many large-breasted women who have undergone breast reductions and subsequently noted significant pain relief. Yet this is a benefit that cannot be guaranteed. Mastectomy is virtually never done for pain relief, since the results are too unpredictable.

WHAT I'D TELL MY DAUGHTER

- Breast pain is common and rarely associated with malignancy.
- Breast pain associated with a lump should be reported to a physician.
- Localized breast pain that seems to be increasing in intensity should be reported to a physician.

CHAPTER SEVEN

Abnormal Mammograms: Calcifications and Densities

OCCASIONALLY, A WOMAN'S SCREENING MAMMOGRAM will show a change from a prior view, despite her being asymptomatic. With these women, additional evaluation is required; further diagnostic evaluation will indicate whether the variations can be safely observed and the patient returned to either a six-month or one-year follow-up.

However, in about 10 percent of cases the difference is of sufficient concern that a biopsy is necessary to make an accurate diagnosis. Two possible changes may have occurred. The most common is the development of new calcifications within the breast; the other is newly revealed areas of increased density.

CALCIFICATIONS

Calcifications are simply deposits of calcium that show up as white dots on a mammogram. Normally, the calcium that circulates in the bloodstream will end up in the bones, but it can be deposited in the breast in response to both benign and malignant changes. The mammographer can readily visualize these deposits. It's the pattern of crystals that is so important to the radiologist in determining whether they are associated with a small evolving cancer or are of no consequence and can be ignored.

The vast majority of calcifications are not indicative of a problem. For the most part, benign calcifications are smooth, round, and scattered throughout the breast. Malignant calcifications, on the other hand, typically concentrate in one spot. They are also more likely to be irregular in shape and small in size.

In most cases, it is relatively easy for the mammographer to distinguish between benign and malignant calcifications. Calcifications that appear benign can be ignored. With some patients the pattern is considered to be *probably* benign, but a six-month follow-up is recommended.

When a pattern is suspicious, a core needle biopsy is recommended as the next step (see "Next Step: Options for Biopsy" on page 47).

DENSITIES

The second common change on the screening mammogram, usually prompting a biopsy, is a new density in the breast. A density is basically an accumulation of tissue that produces a distortion that stands out from the surrounding breast tissue.

In some cases, this change forms a starburst (spiculated) shape that is easy for even the inexperienced observer to visualize. More commonly, the pattern is subtle and can only be observed when comparing the present mammographic images with those from the previous year. For this reason, most mammographers insist on having prior mammograms for comparison.

When the radiologist detects a subtle distortion or density on the screening mammogram, the patient will be called back for additional views, along with a diagnostic ultrasound.

The density may or may not contain calcifications. If it does, it's usually easier for the radiologist to decide on the need for a biopsy. In certain lucky patients, additional views will prove that the density is simply caused by overlapping breast tissue and the patient can return to yearly screening. When findings are labeled as "probably benign," a six-month follow-up mammogram is recommended.

NEXT STEP: OPTIONS FOR BIOPSY

In the "old days," when the calcifications or density were judged to be suspicious, the surgeon would simply remove the area of concern. Now, thanks to improvements in imaging techniques, an open surgical biopsy is rarely performed.

Instead, the modern approach to diagnosis is with a core needle biopsy, which takes a sample of breast tissue that is about the size of the lead in a pencil or larger. This sample not only allows for a more accurate diagnosis, but if the spot proves to be a cancer, the core biopsy provides additional information on how the cancer might respond to various treatment options (see chapter twenty-two).

Three types of core needle biopsies are used to make a more accurate diagnosis: ultrasound-guided core needle biopsies, stereotactic core needle biopsies, and MRI-guided biopsies. (For a detailed description of each, see the boxes on pages 48–49.)

When the spot on the mammogram is also seen on an ultrasound, ultrasound-guided core needle biopsy is the procedure of choice because it is quick and easy for the patient. However, calcifications are typically not seen on the ultrasound and an alternative approach, a stereotactic core biopsy or, in select cases, an MRI-guided biopsy, is required, when the area of concern is seen only on the MRI.

If the biopsy proves to be benign, the patient returns to yearly mammographic screening. If the biopsy shows a high-risk change or a cancer, the patient should be referred to a breast surgeon (see Appendix III).

With some women the findings on the biopsy do not match those on the mammogram—for example, the pattern on the mammogram was suspicious, but the biopsy comes back as normal breast tissue. This inconsistency is referred to as a discordant biopsy. In those situations, a second biopsy is recommended, or the patient is referred to a breast surgeon for consideration for an open biopsy.

ULTRASOUND-GUIDED CORE NEEDLE BIOPSY

In the ultrasound-guided biopsy procedure the patient lies comfortably on her back (with a pillow under her head). The radiologist uses the ultrasound to locate the areas of concern. Local anesthesia is injected into the breast and a small incision is made in the skin. Using the ultrasound as a guide, a core needle biopsy device is directed to the area of concern. The device takes several tissue samples. After completion of tissue sampling, a small titanium clip is placed to identify the spot where the sample was taken. A simple dressing is then placed over the skin incision.

The procedure takes fewer than twenty minutes and is remarkably well tolerated by most patients.

STEREOTACTIC CORE NEEDLE BIOPSY

A stereotactic biopsy is performed when the spot on the mammogram cannot be visualized on the ultrasound. In this procedure the patient lies facedown on the biopsy table. The breast is then positioned so that it hangs through a hole in the table. Below the table is a mammogram machine mounted on a swivel, which allows the technologist to take digital images from the left and right side of the breast at 15-degree angles from the center.

The information from the two images is fed into a computer, which calculates the exact position for optimal placement of the needle tip. Local anesthesia is then injected and a small incision is made in the skin. The needle is advanced into the breast tissue. The computer directs the needle to the correct position for taking an accurate core tissue sample.

After a few samples are taken, the needle is repositioned to take additional samples. As with the ultrasound biopsy, a small titanium clip is placed to mark the location, the needle is removed, and a dressing is applied.

This procedure takes thirty to sixty minutes to perform and is generally well tolerated. In unusual cases it is not possible to do a stereotactic biopsy. With some women, the spot is not in a location that can be accessed on stereotactic imaging. In other cases, the patient may not be able to tolerate lying facedown on a hard table. In these rare cases, an open surgical biopsy is typically performed to make the diagnosis.

MRI-GUIDED BIOPSY

We now commonly perform screening MRIs in women who are considered to be at high risk for malignancies (see Appendix I) but have no breast symptoms and have a normal clinical exam. When the MRI shows a suspicious finding, an ultrasound is recommended, and sometimes special mammographic views are as well. If the area of concern cannot be visualized in either study, the biopsy is done with MRI guidance.

MRI biopsy is done with the patient lying facedown on a mobile table with her arms stretched forward. After proper positioning, the patient is slid into the MRI tube. An MRI study is performed and the area of concern is identified. The patient then slides back out of the machine for needle positioning.

The breast is then gently compressed in a grid. Using targeting software, the radiologist pinpoints the position of the tumor in relation to its location on the grid. The radiologist makes the proper adjustment for needle position and from there on the procedure is similar to that for a stereotactic biopsy.

WHAT I'D TELL MY DAUGHTER

- Most abnormal mammograms prove not to be cancer.
- Needle biopsy is the procedure of choice to evaluate an area of concern on the mammogram or ultrasound.
- Open surgical biopsy to make the diagnosis of an area of concern on the mammogram is rarely indicated.

CHAPTER EIGHT

Breast Lumps

I AM FREQUENTLY ASKED by my patients, "What is a breast lump?" The confusion is understandable, since by nature breasts are lumpy. In general, we think of a breast lump as a localized prominence in the breast that stands out from normal, surrounding tissue.

Fortunately, most lumps are easy for the patient to detect. Nodules that are smooth, round, and movable are typically benign. Malignant masses are usually hard, irregular, and, in more advanced cases, fixed in place. For these women, the issue is mainly making an accurate diagnosis.

However, distinguishing the more subtle lumps from normal breast tissue can be challenging even for an experienced physician, who may be convinced that the questionable area is simply a variation of the normal breast pattern. Unfortunately, many physicians don't understand that any new focal "area of concern" in the breast merits attention. If a woman can point to a specific area where she perceives a change, a directed ultrasound is indicated.

If the ultrasound is not definitive, a focused mammogram should be performed for women in their thirties. Although we do not advise screening mammograms for this age group, diagnostic mammograms to evaluate new symptoms are perfectly safe. In women forty and over, we opt for a diagnostic mammogram with magnification and compression views to the area. If it has been six months or more since the patient's most recent mammogram, regular whole breast views should be included in the diagnostic workup.

If a lump can be visualized on the ultrasound or mammogram, a core needle biopsy is next. For patients in which the evaluation is completely normal, it is important for the physician to understand the need for close follow-up.

For certain malignancies, such as lobular cancer (also known as "the Devil's Cancer"—see chapter ten), a subtle clinical finding may be the only indicator of a developing problem. For this reason we follow up on such patients with additional physical examination at two-, four-, and six-month intervals. A menstruating woman is advised to return five to ten days after the onset of her period. This approach has proven to be effective in avoiding a delayed diagnosis and has been much appreciated by my patients.

For some women a more aggressive approach is indicated. In patients forty and over who have persistent focal symptoms despite a negative workup, a diagnostic MRI should be considered as an additional option. For those in whom the MRI is normal, the likelihood of a hidden cancer is remote.

With all the advances in imaging technology, it is now rare to do an open surgical biopsy to make the diagnosis of a "hidden" breast cancer.

MAKING THE DIAGNOSIS— AS IT WAS YEARS AGO

Incredible progress has been made—not just in detecting breast cancers at an early stage, but also in how we go about making the diagnosis. Years ago when I was in residency training, we did a "traditional" one-step approach: The patient with a lump would sign a consent form allowing the surgeon to do a mastectomy if the pathologist determined during surgery that the area of concern was cancer. We told our patient that if the lump proved to be benign, she would wake up with a small

Band-Aid–like dressing. If, instead, it was cancer, she would find a large dressing with drainage tubes coming out of her chest.

Understandably, this was a hard concept to explain to a young woman who almost certainly did not have cancer. One case stands out as a reminder of just how frustrating this was in "the old days."

THE PATIENT WHO WAS SCARED AWAY

Monique was a twenty-one-year-old foreign exchange student I met during my surgical residency. She showed up at our clinic with a small mass in her left breast. She was alone and clearly apprehensive about being in a breast clinic in a foreign country. Even worse, a young and relatively inexperienced surgical resident was seeing her.

After introducing myself and asking a few questions, I did a careful exam. She had a marble-sized lump in the center of her left breast that was smooth, round, and very movable. I could tell with almost complete certainty that it was not cancer. I also knew in my heart that having her sign a consent form for mastectomy was the wrong thing to do.

At the time I was just a junior surgical resident. Before discussing options with the patient, I asked the chief of surgery for permission to remove the lump without having her sign the standard consent form.

His response sent chills down my spine: "That is not the way we do it here." His tone clearly implied that if I wanted to continue my residency training, I had no choice but to have her sign the consent form.

I went back to the exam room feeling anything but comfortable. Monique appeared to be so vulnerable. I tried to explain to her that in the United States we require a woman to sign a consent form for a possible mastectomy before taking her to surgery to remove a breast mass. I emphasized the probability that her lump being cancer was probably one in a million.

As soon as I mentioned the word "mastectomy," her mind seemed to go blank. I could tell she was not listening to anything else I said. Tears welled in her eyes. She simply turned and walked away. I never saw her again.

DIFFERENT KINDS OF BREAST LUMPS

Most breast lumps will prove to be benign. The younger the woman, the more likely it will not be cancer. However, new nodules in women over forty should be managed with the assumption that they are cancer until proven otherwise. Breast lumps can be divided into two basic categories: cystic and solid.

Breast Cysts

Breast cysts are fluid-filled sacs found mostly in women between the ages of forty and fifty, though they do appear in all age groups. Most cysts do not form lumps and are only detected on breast imaging. Except for the rare cyst that does not have typically benign features on imaging, the majority can be ignored if they do not form a lump.

Of those that can be felt by the patient, most are easily managed and present no risk. One of the truly rewarding events in my practice occurs when a patient has an obvious tender mass, which on ultrasound proves to be smooth, round, and fluid-filled, but, when the mass is aspirated with a needle under ultrasound guidance, the lump completely disappears—along with the woman's fears. These are among the most appreciative patients in my practice.

In rare instances, the cyst is not smooth and round but has some irregular features. These cysts require clinical judgment, but if there is any concern about the possibility of malignancy, a core needle biopsy (see chapter seven) must be done to remove the entire cyst wall.

In other cases, the cyst will recur following repeated aspirations, and a core needle biopsy should also be done to remove the recurrent cyst.

Open biopsy for a cyst without some kind of tissue diagnosis is no longer a common procedure. If surgical removal is advised in the absence of a previous core biopsy, a second opinion should be obtained.

Solid Breast Lumps

Fibroadenoma: Benign

As previously noted, benign breast lumps are usually smooth, round, and mobile. As with any lump, the ultrasound exam is key to making an accurate diagnosis. The most common benign solid breast mass is the fibroadenoma. How we treat women with this suspected condition illustrates our general approach to breast lumps that are thought to be benign.

Young women with breast lumps often show up in my office with a bored expression and an anxious mother. The daughters seem to know intuitively that the overwhelming probability is that their lump is not cancer. Thank God for moms, though, because despite the odds, sometimes a lump in a young woman will be malignant—as was the case of Michelle in chapter one who was only twenty-one when she discovered her lump.

However, in most cases, my young patients felt their nodule by chance as opposed to discovering it in their monthly self-exam. Usually the patient was aware of the problem weeks before telling her mom, hoping it would just go away.

On physical examination, the lump typically meets all the criteria for being benign—and the ultrasound shows a round or oval mass with smooth edges. The inside is gray to white in contrast to the interior of a cyst, which is black.

A small fibroadenoma can be safely observed as long as the patient is willing to come back at regular intervals or return immediately if there are signs of growth. When there is doubt about the diagnosis, or the family is anxious, an ultrasound-guided core needle biopsy (see chapter seven) typically confirms the diagnosis.

Once a benign diagnosis has been established, the pressure is off. Elective surgical removal can be performed if desired. Knowing that the spot is benign allows the surgeon to remove it with a small cosmetic incision on the border of the areola (the pigmented tissue surrounding the nipple), in the armpit, or in the skin fold below the breast (inframammary fold). There is no need to do the incision directly over the mass if a benign diagnosis has been established.

Cystosarcoma Phyllodes (CSP): Low-Grade Malignancy

Phyllodes tumors of the breast are unusual. Though considered malignant, they are curable in most cases. On examination they can look much like a fibroadenoma, which is one reason we prefer to do a core needle biopsy before removing a suspected fibroadenoma. The one clue that a lump may be a phyllodes tumor is rapid growth. When a patient notes that her lump has increased in size over the past several months, a phyllodes tumor should be suspected.

Again, a core needle biopsy makes the diagnosis. These tumors require complete surgical excision, which includes a thin rim of normal breast tissue. Failure to completely remove the tumors sets the stage for recurrence, so doing the surgery right the first time is the key to success. It takes a surgeon who is experienced in dealing with challenging breast problems to deal with cases of CSP.

If a cystosarcoma phyllodes proves to be malignant, patients are typically referred to both a medical and a radiation oncologist, although chemotherapy is not usually given and radiation is of limited benefit. Wide removal with the rim of normal breast tissue is the treatment of choice.

Next Steps for Possibly Malignant Solid Lumps

Solid lumps that are clinically suspicious are common in our practice. They are typically hard, non-mobile, and painless. After a careful exam

FIBROCYSTIC DISEASE: NOT A DISEASE

During the early years of my practice we did not have ultrasound, and mammography was in its infancy. Core needle biopsies were primitive and clumsy and used sparingly, primarily to diagnose larger breast cancers.

The vast majority of biopsies in the early 1970s were still being done by surgically removing the entire breast mass. The most common diagnosis of a surgically removed breast lump was "fibrocystic disease."

Back then we did not have the tools to evaluate the nature of a lump without doing an open biopsy. The decision to do such a biopsy was based primarily on whether or not we could feel a distinct mass. An anxious patient would often prompt us to be more aggressive about surgical removal.

All of the removed lumps were sent to the pathologist. In many cases the pathologist gave us a specific diagnosis, such as fibroadenoma or invasive breast cancer. However, it happened frequently that a specific diagnosis could not be made. Rather than calling the excised material normal breast tissue, it was commonly referred to as fibrocystic disease—when in fact it was just a variant of normal breast tissue.

We now substitute the term "fibrocystic changes" to imply a benign condition noted on core needle biopsy. Once the biopsy establishes the diagnosis of a fibrocystic condition, an open biopsy can usually be avoided.

of the breast and armpit, an ultrasound is ordered, along with a diagnostic mammogram.

The next step, once again, is a core needle biopsy using an ultrasound for guidance. Several samples are taken and a small titanium tissue marker is placed in the center of the mass. The "cores" are sent to pathology for analysis.

The challenge with suspicious breast lumps is making the diagnosis without delay. All too often in my practice I see a patient who has detected a small lump in her breast and her physician told her not to worry. The following is a list of common statements by physicians that should be ignored by patients:

- You're too young to get breast cancer.
- Don't worry; it doesn't run in your family.
- Your mammogram was normal, so it can't be cancer.
- It's just hormonal changes, or it's just fibrocystic disease.
- Breast cancer doesn't cause breast pain.
- You need an open biopsy to make the diagnosis.

Women who suspect a breast lump must be on guard. This is a classic situation in which the woman must be better informed than the average physician, who often doesn't have the time or experience to properly address her concerns.

When a woman suspects a lump, she must tell her physician that she insists on a directed ultrasound and a diagnostic mammogram if needed. If there are abnormal findings, she must demand a core biopsy. If the workup is negative, she should require follow-up visits two, four, and six months after the ultrasound. If there are still questions, she must insist on referral to a breast surgeon.

MAKING A DIAGNOSIS UNDER REAL-LIFE CONDITIONS

Janine found a small nodular prominence in her left breast. She was twenty-eight at the time and was planning her wedding.

On exam, I could feel her lump and it had all the features of a fibroadenoma. The ultrasound appearance was consistent with that diagnosis. She was in a rush and did not have time for a fine needle biopsy.

I explained that the overwhelming odds were that it was a fibroadenoma and could be safely followed. She promised to see me again soon after returning from her honeymoon.

One month later our reminder system indicated that she had not made a follow-up appointment. Our office made a call. I saw her the following day. On exam, her lump seemed slightly more prominent. A biopsy showed an infiltrating ductal cancer. She elected to have both breasts removed and immediate reconstruction. In addition, two of her lymph nodes were positive for metastatic breast cancer—meaning the original cancer had spread.

Janine underwent a course of chemotherapy and tolerated it quite well. One day during chemo she appeared in my office wearing a shocking pink wig. When I think back on Janine's case, a picture of the two of us comes to mind: Janine, with her bald head, and me wearing her flamboyant pink wig.

She is now a twenty-year survivor. She serves as an excellent reminder of how important it is to detect breast cancer early in young women. A longer delay in her case could have led to a less joyous outcome.

WHAT I'D TELL MY DAUGHTER

- Most breast lumps in young women are not cancer.
- Persistent breast lumps require a physician exam.
- Ultrasound should be performed on new breast lumps in young women. Diagnostic mammograms should be done in addition to ultrasound in women forty and older.
- Core needle biopsy is the procedure of choice for making the diagnosis of a solid lump.

CHAPTER NINE

Nipple Discharge

Though nipple discharge is less common than breast pain, it remains one of the symptoms that often brings women to our breast care center. In most cases, the discharge is not caused by cancer. It is fairly easy to determine its significance by asking a few simple questions.

The first question is, "Does the discharge come out spontaneously, or only when you squeeze your nipples?" For reasons unclear to me, many women are under the impression that squeezing the breast and nipples is part of the normal process of breast self-exam.

When a woman tells me she notes the discharge only when squeezing the breast, I tell her the first thing to do is stop squeezing. As it turns out, most women, whether previously pregnant or not, are able to get a drop or more of fluid with vigorous squeezing. But this type of discharge is normal. In most instances the discharge stops when the forceful pressure stops.

The second question is, "What does the discharge look like?" In most cases she will say the discharge is white, green, or other light colors, and I respond that this is of no concern.

If a woman says that it is dark in color, like old blood, or clear, like water, it could be associated with an underlying malignancy.

The clinical exam is just as important as the history. One of the major indicators that we could be dealing with a more serious breast condition is when the discharge is obvious with *gentle* squeezing of the breast. When it's difficult to reproduce the discharge on clinical exam, the odds of it being related to cancer are markedly reduced.

Another clue that suggests a more serious underlying condition is when the discharge is limited to one spot in the nipple. Each breast has ten to fifteen major ducts, the tubes that transport milk to the nipple. When I compress the nipple I look carefully to determine the source of the discharge. If it comes from several ducts, I can be almost certain it is not associated with a malignancy.

Conversely, if the discharge comes from a single duct, a biopsy will likely be required. Nipple discharges associated with a hidden malignancy nearly always come from a single milk duct. In such cases a more detailed evaluation is mandatory.

We make certain that every patient seen in our center with a new nipple discharge has an updated mammogram. If there is even the slightest concern that a discharge may be associated with an underlying breast problem, we do a diagnostic mammogram and ultrasound to look for calcifications or other breast changes. Of course if an area of concern is noted, we perform a biopsy.

The second test that helps us determine the significance of discharge is the breast ultrasound. Often, the ultrasound will visualize an enlarged duct that contains a small mass. An ultrasound-guided core needle biopsy (see chapter seven) would almost always provide a specific diagnosis.

When the mammogram and ultrasound are negative but the discharge persists, an open surgical procedure is usually the next step. The challenge for the surgeon is to make certain the proper duct is removed—and this can be a problem, especially if the discharge is intermittent.

In cases of suspicious discharge, doctors commonly order a special X-ray study of the breast. Called a ductogram, the procedure is simply a study that outlines the internal structure of the breast duct. The procedure involves the placement of a small tube into the discharging duct. A contrast material is gently injected into the opening. Afterward, we do a breast X-ray, and the duct typically lights up, looking much like a branching tree with no leaves.

Normal ducts are smooth and round. When an abnormal growth causes the discharge, it typically shows up as a round or irregular mass that fills or blocks the duct. If the ductogram is completely normal, the patient can be safely observed. However, in some cases, the duct system is not adequately visualized, which usually means surgical removal is the next step.

In our center we prefer to do the ductogram on the morning of surgery. This avoids the problem of not finding the duct on a second attempt. After injecting the contrast material the radiologist injects a drop or two of blue dye to make it more visible to the surgeon. The entire duct, which is often an inch or more in length, is removed and sent to the pathologist.

In the majority of cases, the cause of the discharge is not associated with a malignancy—and thus removal of the discharging duct is curative. The most common cause of spontaneous nipple discharge is a small growth within the duct that is referred to as a papilloma, which is almost always benign. There are other causes of discharge for nipple discharge that are non-cancerous in origin—and all are cured with the removal of the discharging duct.

In approximately 5 percent of cases the discharge is caused by cancer and additional surgery is required. When the discharge is not associated with a breast mass or suspicious changes on the mammogram, the malignancy is almost always detected when it is small and the prognosis is excellent.

Although most cases of nipple discharge are easy to sort out, there are some in which it is difficult to determine the cause. A typical example is a woman who notes what appears to be a spontaneous discharge that looks like old blood, which seems to be coming out of a single duct. Episodes of discharge may occur for a few days and then disappear for weeks. With these patients, the discharge is often gone by the time she sees the doctor. It is common for the woman to bring in her bra, which has spots that resulted from her episodes of spontaneous discharge.

Yet even with intermittent discharge it is common to have a completely normal physician exam and normal breast imaging. In the past we simply followed up with these patients at regular intervals and instructed them to return immediately when the discharge recurred.

Now we have a more effective approach for clarifying the problem of such discharge. If a patient's history is suggestive of a possible malignancy and the workup is completely normal, I recommend an MRI of the breast. When the MRI is normal, I explain to the patient that for practical purposes we can assume she does not have cancer. We continue to keep a watchful eye, but I have yet to see or hear of a case in which the MRI missed cancer as a cause of nipple discharge.

WHAT I'D TELL MY DAUGHTER

- Be concerned about a discharge that occurs on its own without squeezing.

- Any nipple discharge that occurs without squeezing should be evaluated by a physician. (This includes spots on one's bra, even if discharge is not visible.)

- Spontaneous discharge that is bloody or clear is of high concern. Discharge that is white, green, or other colors is rarely associated with a malignancy.

Uncommon but Perilous Breast Problems

CHAPTER TEN

Infiltrating Lobular Cancer: The Devil's Cancer

WHILE EARLY DETECTION PROTOCOLS work for the majority of women, they, like most things in life, are not perfect. One of the most frustrating situations in my practice occurs when a woman who has consistently followed recommended guidelines is diagnosed with a large, advanced breast cancer.

Although this is a rare event, there's one type of malignancy that can be almost impossible to detect before it reaches the size of a large lemon. The proper medical name is infiltrating lobular cancer, but we refer to it as the Devil's Cancer.

The majority of breast cancers arise in the ducts, tubes that connect the milk-producing glands to the nipple. The malignancies that begin here are called infiltrating ductal cancers. They are typically easy to diagnose on screening mammograms long before they grow to the size where a lump can be felt.

Lobular cancers, however, start in the milk-producing glands themselves. Generally, these tumors behave like ductal cancers and are easily detected as well. However, for reasons that are not well understood, the occasional lobular cancer grows to a large size without being detectable on the mammogram or by physical examination. Not only are they difficult to detect at an early stage, but they are also unpredictable in their behavior. Some are very aggressive and resistant to standard treatments. Others are somewhat less aggressive, and have a good prognosis, even when the diagnosis is delayed.

HOW THE DEVIL'S CANCER TAKES HOLD

Diana was serious about following early detection guidelines. She was a single mom raising two young children. She started mammographic screening at age forty and continued on a yearly basis. She was also faithful about doing her monthly self-exam. In addition, her primary care physician examined her on a twelve-month basis. In short, she was a poster child for early detection.

As was her habit, she had her yearly mammogram, followed by her clinical exam, shortly after her forty-seventh birthday. Everything seemed normal.

Two months later, she noticed a pain in her right breast. When it persisted, she made an appointment to see her doctor. The physical examination was completely negative and, since her recent mammogram was also negative, she was advised to "keep an eye on it" and report any changes.

Another two months went by. And then, while she was drying off after a shower, she noticed that the right breast seemed to be larger than the left, and the nipple looked as if it were being pulled into the underlying tissue. She called her doctor and was told to see me immediately.

She came in the next day. Sure enough, I saw that the right breast was enlarged, with a markedly different shape than the other. The entire central and upper area felt firm compared to the opposite side. But still there was no distinct mass.

Hers was a typical presentation for the Devil's Cancer. We did a core needle biopsy that day, and two days later the pathologist confirmed my suspicions.

A breast MRI was performed a few days later. A large area was seen in the right breast and was highly suggestive of an advanced breast tumor. The radiologist estimated the cancer to be more than two inches in diameter. She also noted several enlarged lymph nodes in her armpit (axilla).

Her case was presented to our weekly tumor board and the recommendation was to do a mastectomy first, along with removal of the suspicious lymph nodes. This treatment would be followed by a course of chemo, then radiation.

The pathologist's exam of the mastectomy confirmed the presence of a large infiltrating lobular cancer. The specimen contained seventeen lymph nodes, and eleven of these contained metastatic cancer. Her malignancy fell into the category of a locally advanced cancer, which typically is associated with a poor prognosis.

After recovery from surgery, Diana underwent a full course of aggressive chemotherapy, followed by a course of radiation to the chest wall.

Diana is now a ten-year survivor. She is living proof that you can beat the odds—even when you present with a large malignancy that involves numerous lymph nodes. She has become one of our support volunteers. Her goal is to provide inspiration and hope to other women who have been diagnosed with an advanced breast cancer.

THE DEVIL'S CANCER ON THE ATTACK

Maria (not her real name) had a more complicated situation, though she was almost as consistent as Diana in following early detection guidelines.

At age fifty-six she had her yearly mammogram, and then a clinical exam, and both were completely normal. Several months later she returned to her physician with a new pain in the upper left breast. In view of eventual developments, it was surprising that once again the physical exam was normal, and even an ultrasound of the suspicious area showed nothing.

Maria was advised to return to the breast clinic in two months. But with the pain now gone, as well as the fact that she was changing insurance plans, she cancelled her appointment. Instead, she had a follow-up mammogram at her usual one-year interval. No symptoms were noted at the time, and once again the physical breast examination was normal.

Many months later, however, she discovered a mass the size of a ping-pong ball in her left armpit. She also felt a vague prominence in the upper outer left breast in the same area where she had first noticed pain.

Our physical exam showed a highly suspicious mass in the armpit, typical of a metastatic lymph node. Also, there was a firm fullness in the left breast, but still with no distinct lump. This time an ultrasound of the area was suggestive of a malignancy. A biopsy of both the breast mass and the lump in the armpit showed infiltrating lobular cancer.

Maria subsequently underwent mastectomy, chemotherapy, and radiation. She was found to have a large cancer in the mastectomy specimen, along with multiple metastatic lymph nodes.

Maria did remarkably well with her treatments and remained in good health for the next three years, at which time she noted lower back pain. Initially she suspected she had strained her back while lifting something, but the pain progressed.

Shortly thereafter, she was seen by her oncologist. A bone scan revealed extensive metastasis to the bone. She was started on a second course of chemo and had an excellent response. Though Maria remains optimistic, she understands the long-term odds are against her.

Fortunately, Devil's Cancer accounts for only 10 to 13 percent of all breast cancers. For the vast majority of patients, standard early detection protocols work, and diagnostic delays are rare.

It is difficult explaining to the small percentage of women who are diagnosed with advanced lobular cancers why the mammogram missed their malignancies. Wanting an explanation, they frequently ask, "Why did the mammogram let me down?" There is no easy answer to this question. When pressed for an explanation, I start the conversation by explaining how different types of breast cancers have remarkably different growth patterns. Cancers of lobular origin often behave differently from most ductal cancers, though they still have some similarities.

Ductal cancers, like all such malignancies, start with one wayward cell that breaks through the body's control mechanisms and starts growing out of control on its own. The rapidly dividing cells stick together and form a ball of cells. With continued growth, the ball reaches the size where it can be easily detected on the mammogram and/or felt as a mass.

The cells in lobular cancers, however, unlike most of those in ductal cancers, tend to be less inclined to stick together. Rather than forming a ball of cells, they often develop into what can be described as a cobweb-like structure. The cancer simply grows out in multiple, single-file directions and into the surrounding breast tissue rather than forming a distinct mass, or ball. As the cancer infiltrates the nearby tissue, the thickness of the web increases. With a thickening web, the spaces between branches of the web get progressively smaller. Eventually the web coalesces to form a solid mass of cancer cells. As a result, it often seems that the breast becomes distorted in size and shape overnight.

Whatever the explanation, the conclusion is the same. As yet, we have not developed a successful strategy for detecting a malignancy with this type of growth pattern when it is small and early in its development.

Progress is being made, however, and there is reason for hope in the near future. One recent advance has been to understand how cancers can hide in women with dense breasts (see chapter fourteen). As stated earlier, ultrasound and MRI are very effective in detecting small malignancies that cannot be seen on the screening mammogram. It is likely that as more women with dense breasts undergo additional screening, more small cancers, including those of lobular origin, will be detected earlier in their development.

Two recent advances in breast imaging may also facilitate early detection of these stubborn cancers. We know that the breast MRI is more effective than the mammogram in detecting small tumors. A major problem with the MRI is cost. Research is now being done to determine the effectiveness of an Ultra-Fast MRI designed for the purpose of screening asymptomatic women. If costs can be brought under control, this could prove to be a major advance in our early detection efforts.

Also, a new breast-imaging technique is being developed at the Mayo Clinic. According to early reports, this new technology can almost quadruple the detection of early cancers in women with dense breasts, catching tumors while they're still very small. The technique is referred to as molecular breast imaging, or MBI. The procedure calls for the injection of a radioactive substance (low-dose radiation) that concentrates in small cancers. After injection, the breast is visualized on a screen and tiny cancers show up as obvious hot spots.

These techniques could be major advancements in our quest for early detection of the Devil's Cancer.

CHAPTER ELEVEN

Inflammatory Breast Cancer: The Silent Killer

A S WORRISOME AS the Devil's Cancer is to doctors, inflammatory breast cancer is right on par—except this is a rare malignancy that can quietly affect women before anyone notices.

Inflammatory breast cancer (IBC) is not only the most aggressive type of breast tumor, it is also the most elusive when it comes to making a diagnosis. Often referred to as the "silent killer," IBC has too often spread to other parts of a woman's body before a diagnosis is even made.

Much like invasive lobular cancer, the cells in IBC often do not form a lump that can be felt or seen on imaging. One of the early indications that a woman has a hidden inflammatory breast cancer is the development of breast redness that looks like an early breast infection. However, the absence of a fever is one clue that the redness is not related to an infection.

Not only is IBC difficult to diagnose, it is also difficult to define. When I started my training, the term IBC was restricted to cases in which the redness involved most of the breast. To meet this older criterion for IBC, physicians required extensive skin thickening and enlargement of the lymph nodes in the armpit.

INFLAMMATORY BREAST CANCER—AS IT ONCE WAS

I saw my first case of IBC several months after I started my private practice in 1973. Jane (not her real name) was twenty-eight when she first noted redness in the center of her right breast—a discoloration that seemed to spread rapidly.

Her physician assumed she had an infection and started her on an antibiotic. To her surprise, a week later the breast seemed heavy and swollen. The nipple appeared to be flattening compared to the nipple on the left. Jane was given a second, more potent antibiotic, but the swelling and redness continued to progress.

By the time I saw her, about three weeks into treatment, the right breast was almost twice the size of the left. The skin had the appearance of an orange peel, and I could feel enlarged lymph nodes in her armpit that were suspicious of metastatic breast cancer.

Her mammogram showed skin thickening but no visible mass. On that first visit, we did an old-fashioned, spring-loaded needle biopsy of the breast and a punch biopsy, in which a cutting tool is used to sample skin changes on the surface; the tool removes a small 2mm-to-4mm disc of breast skin. Both showed cancer.

Adding the biopsy finding to the clinical picture, we knew that hers was a classic example of inflammatory breast cancer. We did not know then what we know now about IBC—and our treatment in cases of advanced IBC were not very effective.

Over the following decades, the definition of what constitutes an inflammatory breast cancer has continued to evolve. Even now it is common in our tumor boards for experienced physicians to argue back and forth as to whether a newly diagnosed breast cancer meets the "true definition" of an IBC or if it is just a case of an aggressive breast cancer with associated skin redness.

My impression is that the term IBC is now being applied to most aggressive breast cancers that cause redness of the overlying skin. And the general consensus seems to be that redness is a sign of a malignancy's more hostile behavior and a poorer prognosis. Thus, more vigorous therapy is required to treat patients with skin redness than would be for breast cancer of the same size without the redness.

Although progress is being made in standardizing the terminology from the physician's perspective, things are still very confusing from the patient's point of view.

ONE WOMAN'S FIGHT FOR IBC EDUCATION

The issue of patient frustration became obvious to me after I gave a lecture on breast cancer care to a large group of women. The talk went well, and the audience was very enthusiastic.

As is commonly the case, after the lecture many women approached me with questions and stories. As the audience was leaving, one woman came to me with a smile on her face and politely said, "You doctors don't know anything about IBC."

Rather than getting defensive, I asked her to explain. "Mary" told me she had just finished her second course of chemotherapy. She was now in remission, but she was still concerned about her long-term prognosis.

As she related to me, her story started two years earlier when she noted a patch of redness on her left breast. Initially, she was not concerned, but the area of redness expanded rapidly. Over the next several weeks she was seen by multiple physicians, all of whom reassured her that she had a breast infection that was not responding to standard therapy.

She was given several courses of different antibiotics with no result. One morning while taking a shower, she felt a lump in her armpit. She called her physician, who referred her to a surgeon. By this time the redness extended to most of her breast, and her skin now looked like the peel of an orange.

A biopsy of the lymph node was positive. She was referred to an oncologist, who quickly started her on chemo. Two years after she'd finished the first course, the cancer reappeared in her bones, and a second course of chemo was begun.

Her frustration was easily understood. Like most patients, she assumed that if the diagnosis had been made on an earlier doctor's visit, her prognosis would have been more favorable.

She also pointed out to me that not one single doctor even considered the diagnosis of IBC. It was not until she was seen by a surgeon that the clinical diagnosis was made. Her frustration led her to do a web search to learn more about IBC. What she found was a large number of women with similar stories. Their diagnoses were typically delayed for weeks or months because their physicians were seemingly unaware that redness of the breast could be an early sign of an aggressive cancer.

Until recently, the majority of people had never heard the term "inflammatory breast cancer." Public awareness changed dramatically in May 2006, following a television interview and special report on Seattle's KOMO News with a mother whose teenage daughter was similarly diagnosed. Again, diagnostic delays gave the girl's cancer time to spread to other parts of her body.

A plea was made: Women should report any new skin redness of the breast to the doctor and, when necessary, explain that they are concerned about the possibility of IBC. The interview struck a chord with the public and millions of women who watched the video on their computers.

From a public education perspective, this was a major accomplishment—but it did have its downsides. The one line that seemed to stick in the public's mind was that the first indication of IBC could be a small red spot on the breast that looks like a bug bite. We started receiving a large number of calls from women who were concerned that they might have an early case of IBC. Not only were their tensions at an all-time high, but the prevailing attitude indicated these women knew more about IBC than we did. They'd already been warned that doctors didn't know much about the malady and in all likelihood would not take their concerns seriously.

As a result, we had to spend more time and do more testing to reassure them that they did not have cancer. IBC is a relatively rare form of breast cancer, and, not surprisingly, we did not see a single case of it during this period of high anxiety.

Eventually, the hysteria subsided. The good news from all the media publicity and various blogs was that both the public and physicians became more aware of the relationship between redness of the breast and the possibility of an underlying breast cancer.

Even with a high level of knowledge, however, it is still difficult to make the diagnosis of IBC as quickly as we do with other types of breast cancer. Over time I have developed a step-by-step approach to making the diagnosis in as timely a manner as I think is possible.

One of my first recommendations for women who have what appears to be a simple bug bite is to observe it for a day or two. In most cases the redness will disappear within these few days. If the redness persists for more than two days, the patient should be seen by her doctor or me in the clinic as soon as possible. Fortunately, the vast majority of patients with breast redness will not have a hidden breast cancer.

Most of our patients with a short history of redness will have an otherwise normal exam and normal breast imaging. In these cases, all that is needed is a seven-to-ten-day course of antibiotics and a return office visit in one week. Usually, the redness will have disappeared by then. However, these patients should still be followed for several months because of the unlikely possibility that they do have IBC and that the inflammation has just temporarily gone away.

If the redness does not go away completely, or if it recurs, the patient should be referred to a surgeon. My first step after reviewing the history and doing a careful clinical exam is to ultrasound the breast. If I see an area of concern, I do an ultrasound-guided aspiration. Usually I can get at least a few drops of fluid, which is then sent for culture to determine whether any bacteria are present. I also have the pathologist evaluate the fluid for the presence of malignant cells.

If nothing is seen on the ultrasound, I do what I refer to as a "blind needle aspiration." A needle is directed into the breast tissue below the area of redness, and again a few drops of fluid are collected and sent for further studies. If, after these initial steps, the evaluation is still inconclusive, the patient is placed on a new antibiotic and scheduled to return in one week.

If the redness persists on the second visit, the next step is to do a core needle biopsy (see chapter seven) of the underlying breast tissue. In patients with more advanced skin changes, we also do a skin punch biopsy (which removes a small circle of skin to be sent to the pathologist for analysis; see "Inflammatory Breast Cancer—As It Once Was" on page 74) on the skin in the area of the redness. In addition, we perform an ultrasound on the armpit, looking for suspicious lymph nodes. If suspicious lymph nodes are found, a tissue sample is taken with either a fine needle or a core needle.

In my experience, this aggressive approach to making the diagnosis is highly successful in the majority of cases of IBC. However, with a few patients, these steps still fail to produce an accurate picture, a fact that must be kept in mind. After giving the patient the good news that her biopsy was negative, it is important to follow her over the next several months. When symptoms progress or reappear, consideration should be given to repeat core biopsies covering larger areas of the breast than were done initially.

In my entire career, I have seen only two cases of IBC in which the diagnosis could *only* be made with an open surgical biopsy. This option is a last resort—and only when all other approaches fail. I assume that now, with modern biopsy techniques, an open biopsy will rarely, if ever, be required for future diagnoses.

In contrast to the multiple problems involved in making an accurate diagnosis, the treatment recommendations for IBC have finally become standardized. In the old days, soon after the disease was identified, the surgeon would typically do a mastectomy. After recovering from surgery, the patient was sent to a medical oncologist for chemotherapy. Following chemo, she was turned over to a radiation oncologist for chest wall radiation.

Now the order is reversed. The surgeon is typically the one who makes the clinical diagnosis of IBC. Once it is made, the patient is sent directly to the medical oncologist for chemotherapy. In most cases, the chemo is highly effective in reducing the size of the cancer, which makes it easier for the surgeon to remove the breast without the need to transfer skin from other parts of the body to close the gap. The third steps is to radiate the chest wall following mastectomy.

Yet sometimes the tumor is more advanced and less responsive to chemo; in these unusual cases, breast radiation further shrinks the breast for an easier mastectomy.

The breast cancer specialists at the prestigious MD Anderson Cancer Center in Houston, Texas, were the first physicians to recommend this three-step approach for the treatment of IBC. A recent report from their clinic indicates that approximately one-fourth of the IBC patients they see for a second opinion have not been advised to undergo what is now considered this standard approach.

It's a disturbing finding. Unfortunately, it indicates that significant numbers of women with IBC are receiving inadequate treatment, which translates into a lower probability of survival.

If a woman who has recently been diagnosed with IBC has any questions about the appropriateness of her treatment, she should consider getting a second opinion—quickly—from a breast center with experience in treating women with this rare malignancy.

CHAPTER TWELVE

Paget's Disease of the Nipple

THERE IS ONE DISTINCT warning sign that indicates the presence of a potentially curable breast cancer. Failure to perceive the significance of this early indicator can have major adverse consequences. The chief warning sign is a subtle change in the appearance of the nipple.

PAGET'S DISEASE

Paget's disease of the nipple is a condition in which cancer starts evolving just below the surface of the skin. The earliest changes in the appearance of the nipple are often subtle and easily confused with symptoms associated with non-cancerous conditions.

The first indicators of Paget's can be redness and slight tenderness of one nipple. As the cancer grows, the nipple skin develops a scaly appearance, much like what occurs with eczema or other non-cancerous skin conditions. When diagnosis of the disease is delayed, the skin changes become more obvious. Small ulcerations appear in the nipple and can spread to the surrounding areola. If left untreated, the nipple can become completely eroded, while the cancer spreads into the breast.

The classic form of Paget's is a slow-growing cancer, which allows the clinician enough time to make the diagnosis. The challenge for the physician is to make a timely diagnosis while the nipple changes are subtle and consistent with other benign conditions. In my experience, the key to making an early diagnosis is to listen to your patient. My rule is that any time a woman notes a change in appearance or texture in one nipple, she has Paget's disease until proven otherwise. On occasion, I see women who express concern about one nipple when, to me, the appearance is normal. Paget's disease is rare in these cases. I make sure the patient's mammogram is up to date and have them return at two, four, and six months. In most cases, the nipple will remain stable, and no other treatment is indicated.

My approach is fairly simple: If a woman comes to our center with a concern about such changes, and on exam I am suspicious of the diagnosis, I do a skin punch biopsy (see chapter eleven) of the nipple on her first visit. The punch biopsy is performed under local anesthesia, takes only a few minutes, and is almost painless. The small tissue sample is sent immediately to the pathologist, and the diagnosis is made in two to three days.

More commonly, I see women with vague changes in the nipple that do not suggest Paget's disease. For them I recommend a ten-day course of over-the-counter hydrocortisone cream to be applied twice daily, with a return visit in two weeks. I have never seen or heard of a case of Paget's of both nipples. If a woman comes to me with similar changes on both sides, I recommend she see a dermatologist.

In most patients, the changes will be much improved or gone by the second office visit. However, these women still need careful observation. If there is any evidence of progression and the nipple changes did not respond to topical treatment, a punch biopsy is required.

Making the diagnosis of Paget's disease is usually easy, but even with this aggressive approach, there can be major challenges—as the following case illustrates.

AN ODD CASE OF PAGET'S DISEASE

At the time of her first visit to our center, Monica, a nurse, was forty-two years old. She told me she was worried that she might have Paget's disease. She had noticed some irritation of the right nipple, and also that it looked different from the left. She applied cortisone cream and in a few days the appearance returned to normal.

Her story caught me by surprise. I would have assumed that she'd cancel her appointment if the appearance returned to normal so quickly. I was even more surprised that she still believed that her symptoms could have been caused by Paget's disease. Her follow-up exam was normal, as was her updated mammogram. I recommended she keep an eye on things and return immediately if she noted changes. Otherwise I would see her at two-, four-, and six-month intervals.

She seemed relieved that I took her symptoms seriously, and she made all three follow-up visits. Her exam remained completely normal and at the time she had no further problems.

On her third exam she'd had her yearly mammogram. The appearance of her nipple had remained stable and the mammogram was reported as normal. At the time of my clinical exam she still had nipple markers adherent to each nipple. The markers are used to clarify the position of the nipple, which makes it easier for the radiologist to interpret the findings on the mammogram. The markers are sticky and must be carefully removed to avoid pain.

When I slowly removed the marker from the right nipple, a small layer of skin came with it. The area where the skin came off appeared irritated and obviously different from the left side. This was a highly unusual finding. A punch biopsy was done during this same visit, and it proved positive for Paget's disease. The standard treatment for Paget's at that time was mastectomy, which was performed a week later without any technical problems.

So despite having had a normal mammogram a week before the surgery, it turned out Monica had guessed right months before the diagnosis. The pathologist found extensive, non-invasive cancer (ductal carcinoma in situ or DCIS) in the mastectomy specimen. Fortunately, Monica was cured by the mastectomy and did not need chemo or radiation.

A GOOD DIAGNOSIS — FROM A DISTANCE

I have never seen Shannon as a patient. In fact, Shannon lives in Ireland. I recently received an email from her, thanking me for saving her life. It is the only case in my career in which I was given credit for a cure without ever seeing the patient.

Shannon was thirty-six when she first noted some "flaking" on the tip of her right nipple. Over a period of several weeks, the spot seemed to be getting worse. Yet the left nipple was completely normal.

She made an appointment to see her primary care doctor, who immediately dismissed it as a common case of dermatitis and told her not to worry. She was upset that her doctor was not taking her concerns seriously. Unsure what to do next, like so many women, she turned to the internet. In less than an hour of research, she was convinced she had Paget's disease.

At a second appointment with her doctor, she mentioned her internet search and explained she was certain she had the disease. Again he told her not to worry, in a tone that suggested she was overreacting.

Increasingly frustrated, but with low expectations, Shannon went back to her computer. During her search, she found the website for the Be Aware Foundation. The goal of the foundation is to inspire women to follow early detection guidelines. One of the free services offered is a monthly email reminder to do breast self-exam. Attached to each email is an article I write on breast health. One piece was on Paget's disease.

After reading my discussion, Shannon knew immediately what to do next. She made a copy of the article and showed it to her doctor, then insisted on an immediate punch biopsy of her nipple, which proved positive for Paget's disease.

In her subsequent email to me she expressed her overwhelming gratitude, and she stated she could now rest assured that her two young children would grow up with a "healthy mum."

Monica's and Shannon's stories show that no two cases of Paget's disease are exactly alike, and, while sometimes it is easy for a woman to detect the condition, it can be hard to convince a physician, as was the case for Shannon. It's not surprising that diagnostic delays are common in women with Paget's disease.

SOMETIMES A WOMAN IS HER BREAST'S BEST FRIEND

A patient, whom I'll call Donna, was in her early sixties when she noted changes in her left nipple. Over the next three years she was seen by ten different physicians, including two dermatologists.

In frustration, she called a family member on the East Coast who was a primary care physician. He told her that her symptoms were typical of Paget's disease. Armed with this information, she went back to her dermatologist, who seemed irritated by the information. Again he told her it was nothing to worry about and to continue using the skin ointments that he had prescribed.

In desperation, she decided to drive the extra fifty miles to be seen at our comprehensive breast care center. The diagnosis was obvious. By then the tiny ulcerations in the skin had spread to the surrounding areola. The rest of the clinical exam was normal. We did a skin punch on that visit, and it proved positive for Paget's disease.

Her mammogram revealed extensive calcifications, which meant she needed a mastectomy. The mastectomy specimen showed extensive invasive cancer in the breast, plus two lymph nodes, which also contained metastatic disease.

Because of the advanced state of her malignancy, she was given a course of chemo following surgery. Donna had a hard time with chemo, but she is now doing well. Donna's extensive disease could have been avoided if a punch biopsy had been performed when she first went to her physicians with the changes in her nipple, or if the earlier physicians had taken her concerns seriously.

PAGET'S DISEASE WITH A CINDERELLA ENDING

Pat (her real name), one of my established patients, returned to the office between her regular visits because of subtle skin changes in the tip of one nipple. A skin punch biopsy revealed Paget's disease. Imaging indicated it was localized to the nipple.

She had large breasts that had lost their youthful shape. The nipple and surrounding area were removed, along with a large segment of underlying breast tissue, completely clearing the area of cancer. The remaining breast tissue was rearranged to give her a youthful contour. We then did a reduction on the left breast so it matched the right.

A few months later, my son Justin constructed a new nipple, followed by tattooing to match the normal appearance. After several months of recovery, she was boasting about her newly acquired girlish figure.

Controversies in Breast Care

THE ISSUES IN THIS SECTION provided most of the inspiration for this book. In recent years, so-called experts have radically "changed the game," issuing new breast care guidelines that my years of experience have proven are both false and dangerous. It's difficult to stand by and make no effort to counter public statements that I know will have the potential of causing harm to large numbers of women.

CHAPTER THIRTEEN

The Breast Self-Exam Controversy

THE CONCEPT OF DOING monthly breast self-examination (BSE) seems so logical it's hard to believe any reputable organization would suggest making it optional.

ONE WOMAN'S INTRODUCTION TO BSE

Lisa was invited by a friend to go to the Susan G. Komen Race for the Cure. At the time she was thirty-three. After the run, Lisa and her friend did a tour of the many booths surrounding the main event. Some of the vendors were passing out brochures on health and fitness, and others were handing out goodies to attract the attention of passersby.

That night while watching television, Lisa looked through her goodie bag. One item caught her attention—a pamphlet titled "How to Do Breast Self-Examination." Since she'd never done this before, she decided to give it a try. She was wearing a nightgown at the time, which made it easier.

The left breast seemed normal. But when she probed the right, she felt an area of prominence in the upper area of the breast that was different from the other side.

She was not overly concerned, but the next day she told her friend about her finding. The friend insisted she report it to her doctor. Lisa saw her physician a few days later, with unfortunate results; he insisted her exam was normal and not to worry. Lisa's friend was skeptical about the doctor's recommendation, and told Lisa she needed to see a specialist. The friend gave her my name.

I saw her the next day. She did have a vague prominence on the right breast, but to me it did not feel suspicious. To be on the safe side, however, I did an ultrasound exam. The readout made it immediately evident that a small mass lurked where Lisa felt the "difference." The appearance on ultrasound was suspicious. And indeed, a biopsy was positive for an invasive cancer.

Fortunately, Lisa's malignancy was small and she did not need chemo. The lump was removed as an outpatient procedure, and surgery was followed by a six-week course of radiation. Sixteen years later it's hard to tell which breast had the surgery.

On each of her yearly visits she shows me pictures of her three children. Every time I see her, I am reminded about how easy it was for her to detect a small cancer on her first attempt at self-exam. All it took was a 15-cent brochure to save her life.

Anyone who doubts the overwhelming value of breast self-examination (BSE) should read Lisa's story. This example, and many more like it, has convinced me that BSE can be lifesaving. Teaching women to do the exam with confidence takes time and effort. For years my wife, Jan, who is a registered nurse, taught self-exam classes; her sessions were always full, with a waiting list to get in.

However, this program came to an abrupt halt in early 2008 when the American Cancer Society and, shortly after, the Susan G. Komen organization announced their new guidelines for breast self-examination. Basically both organizations now agree that doing BSE is not recommended. However, the new guidelines state that women should still be *self-aware* and report any change to their doctor.

It takes a committee to come up with recommendations that are this confusing. I can only assume that some group members were for it and some against, so the compromise was to try to have it both ways: in effect saying, *You really don't need to do this exam, but in case you do, watch out for anything suspicious.* How confusing is that?

As a result of the new guidelines, my wife could no longer fill her classes, and within a year all sessions were cancelled. I am convinced that informing the public that self-exams don't work has led to diagnostic delays. Undoubtedly, some delays have resulted in the need for more aggressive treatments and lowered chances of survival.

The most common question I get from patients about this issue is, "Why the change?" The stated explanation is that the advisory committees of both organizations concluded there was insufficient scientific data to prove that doing self-exam saved lives. To support their contention, they pointed to a study done on Chinese factory workers and reported in the *Journal of the National Cancer Institute* in 2002. Half the women were taught to do regular self-exams and the other half were not given any instructions. The group of women who learned to do BSE did not find either smaller or more numerous cancers than the group who were not instructed at all. Worse, the group doing self-exams had more negative (or unnecessary) biopsies.

Apparently the committee was not impressed with similar studies on North American women—*which came to the opposite conclusion*—that women doing breast self-exams were more apt to find malignancies while they were still small, with an increase in survival rates compared to the others.

The reality is that it is almost impossible to design a truly scientific study that isolates BSE as an independent factor in detecting early breast cancer. There are just too many other elements that influence the odds for early detection. Like many of life's important decisions, the choice to do BSE is based primarily on common sense. After all, the exam is free, and it works. It is the only practical, home-based test that can be done on a monthly basis. It is also the only screening method we have for average-risk women under forty who are not yet getting yearly mammograms. Self-exam is just one more layer of protection to bolster a woman's odds of detecting cancer at its earliest stage.

I also believe that Komen and ACS have taken the wrong approach to the issue of too many unnecessary biopsies. I agree with them that this is a problem and should be addressed, but making self-exams optional is not the answer. Radiologic and surgical organizations have well-established guidelines to deal with the issue of unnecessary biopsies. Most lumps detected on self-exam can be followed without biopsy. Open biopsies to make the diagnosis should rarely be performed. Questionable cysts can be aspirated in the office. Likewise, core needle biopsies are an effective way to examine suspicious lesions and provide definite identification.

The public would have been better served if the new guidelines had encouraged women to get a second opinion before scheduling a biopsy (see chapter twenty-three). Women who are cared for by an experienced physician who is well-versed in breast care can expect to have low rates of negative biopsies. What women need is better access to doctors who are experts in deciding when a biopsy is needed and choosing the least traumatic way to make an accurate diagnosis.

Another point made by ACS and Komen in defending their position is that the process of doing BSE causes a great deal of anxiety for women. The reality is that there is no way to eliminate anxiety when it comes to screening for breast cancer. The best approach is to teach women to do self-exam with confidence. Rather than making BSE optional, the focus should be twofold: persuading women to do it in the first place—but also showing them how to do it better.

The challenge here is that there is no general agreement about how teaching should be done. My wife's classes worked well for those women who participated, but most of my patients never found time to get there. We needed a better way to teach BSE, and Karen's story, which follows, inspired me to think differently about how it should be taught.

KAREN'S STORY—THE IDEAL PATIENT

Karen is the ideal patient. She started doing yearly mammograms at age forty and never missed a year. She is also consistent about doing monthly self-exams and does them with confidence.

She sees me every year in January on the same day she gets her mammogram. Every year, for more than a decade, her breast exam and mammogram were normal. Yet a few years ago she returned to the office in June, five months after her usual visit. I asked why she was seeing me at this short interval, and she replied she felt a change in her left breast.

"A lump?" I asked.

"No," she said. "It just feels different."

I examined both breasts, focusing on the area of her concern. To me, everything seemed completely normal. But an ultrasound showed a small irregular mass that was highly suspicious for cancer. Knowing what was seen on the ultrasound, I re-examined the suspicious area.

Even with advance notice from the ultrasound, I could not detect a distinct lump. She could feel it and I couldn't.

It turned out that Karen did have a malignancy and needed a lumpectomy and radiation, but no chemo.

My lesson from Karen's case was obvious: A woman who knows her own anatomy is likely to be better at detecting a small cancer—basically a "change"—than a knowledgeable breast surgeon. Keeping that in mind, I realized we needed to reevaluate how we go about teaching woman to do BSE with confidence.

To date, all the focus has been on finding lumps. Since the breasts are naturally lumpy, or nodular, it's not surprising that most women experience anxiety when learning how to tell the difference between a normal bumpy texture and a lump that requires attention.

Now I tell women to forget the word "lump" and to just focus on the word "normal." The goal for women is to have a clear mental image of "normal," just like Karen did. Once they grasp what is usual for them and do the exam monthly, they are better than the doctor at detecting subtle changes.

Timing—when to start learning to do proper self-exam—is critical. I often ask my patients, "What is the best night of the year to start doing BSE?" I usually get a blank stare. Then I tell them, "Tonight's the night." At first the comment provokes a little chuckle, and then they get it.

The point is, the time to start learning BSE is on the same day you have a good-news mammogram and the physician's exam is also normal—what I'd call "Ground Zero," meaning zero cancer. Once you have a physical understanding of what is "normal," your fingertips will immediately alert your brain if a change is noted. Knowing what to expect, you are the best person in the world to determine whether anything is suddenly different—that perhaps something is growing in your breast.

One of the most difficult aspects of encouraging women to learn BSE is the issue of time. With scant minutes to do proper teaching in an office setting, I decided to make a video that explains in detail how to do a proper self-exam, thus solving at least the time problem (to watch the video, go to beawarefoundation.org/content/Breast-Self -Examination--BSE-.html). A video is a practical solution, as it can be viewed at the patient's convenience and referenced whenever necessary.

A second objective is to motivate women to do the exam monthly. To help them remember, our foundation sends an email reminder on the first of every month. With each email, we also include a short article on breast care issues. Women can sign up for these on the same website as the video. The monthly email is ideal for menopausal women who can select any day of the month to do self-exam. However, the ideal time for a young menstruating woman is five to ten days after the onset of her period. During this interval, estrogen levels are low and the breast is at its least tender and nodular, meaning it is easier to detect any changes that are not related to her menstrual cycle.

FINDING A SMALL BREAST LUMP is a challenge for women of any age. What to do after discovery can be equally baffling. The next step is to locate a doctor who will take your concerns seriously. Diagnostic delays are common, and to avoid them, every woman must have a clear understanding of what needs to be done if, on a BSE, she finds a worrisome area.

If you detect a change in your breast, at minimum an attentive doctor should take a history and do a careful exam. If it has been more than six months since your last mammogram, a new one should scan the suspicious area. If it's been more than a year, both breasts should be imaged, with additional focus on the problem spot. In nearly all cases I recommend doing an ultrasound exam directed to the suspicious area, even when I am almost certain it is not cancer.

Women such as Lisa, Karen, and Michelle—especially Michelle, the young woman from the Introduction whose concerns about a lump were ignored by multiple doctors because "you're too young to have breast cancer"—are forever in the back of my mind. *How many more women will be denied a diagnosis until it's too late?* I often wonder.

When I do see a patient who has found a suspicious spot on her breast, my goal is to get a specific diagnosis and go from there. The next steps are straightforward and described in chapter eight.

With patients for whom the initial exam and diagnostic studies are normal, the next step is to make follow-up arrangements. I typically try to see these women at two-, four-, and six-month intervals to be certain I am not missing something . . . with the advice to return sooner if there is any indication of progression.

As with BSE, peri-menopausal women are more difficult to schedule, since periods are unpredictable. I simply tell the patient, "If your breasts are tender on the day of the next visit, cancel your appointment and reschedule for the following week." This approach works. It provides patients with confidence and reassurance that they are being cared for. Every woman deserves this level of attention.

WHAT I'D TELL MY DAUGHTER

- Start doing breast exams as soon as breast development occurs.
- Start regular monthly self-exams by age twenty-one.
- Menstruating women should do self-exams five to ten days after the onset of their period.
- Go to beawarefoundation.org to see a self-exam video and sign up for monthly reminders.

CHAPTER FOURTEEN

"My Mammogram Was Normal, and Now I'm on Chemo"

P ATIENTS OFTEN TELL ME about a friend who has undergone chemotherapy. As the story goes, the friend found a lump that proved to be cancer, but her recent mammogram had been "completely normal." The story is unnerving, since such an anecdote is typically shared on the same visit when I am giving the patient the results of her own mammogram.

Here an explanation is needed: The mammogram is nothing more than an X-ray of the breast. It is basically a picture in black and white with more than fifty shades of gray.

Unlike a chest X-ray in which organs like the heart are easily identified, a mammogram of the breast looks to the untrained observer like the surface of the moon. However, even an untrained observer can see that some mammograms have a mostly black pattern and in others the display is mostly white. Women with the white pattern are those with dense breasts. About half of my patients fall into this category.

Breasts that appear predominantly black on film are composed mostly of fatty tissue, meaning that women with this makeup are lucky, since for them the mammogram is very effective. The reason for this is straightforward: Breast cancers typically show up as white spots. These spots are easily seen when the background is black. Finding small cancers in fatty breasts is like detecting a lighted match in a dark room. For these fortunate women, usually no other imaging studies are needed.

The situation is reversed in women with dense breasts. With them, mammograms appear mostly white. Not surprisingly, it is a challenge to detect a small white cancer in a predominantly white background. Trying to find these small cancers in women with dense breasts has been described as looking for a snowman in a snowstorm.

Luckily, we now have ultrasound technology, which has a major advantage in detecting small breast cancers in women with dense breasts. Just as with the mammogram, dense breast tissue looks white on the ultrasound. The superiority of this screening is that cancers typically appear black, and thus they stand out against the white background—the reverse of what happens for women with fatty breasts.

Although I am cognizant of the lifesaving benefits of screening mammograms—worldwide studies have proven that this test reduces breast cancer mortality by more than 30 percent—I am also keenly aware of their limitations.

At our center's weekly tumor board conferences, we review all newly diagnosed breast cancers. In the majority of cases the screening mammogram was successful in detecting small and potentially curable breast cancers.

However, it is not unusual to review cases in which the mammogram missed a large tumor. In most of these events, it was the patient who found a lump. The mammogram was normal, but a diagnostic ultrasound showed an obvious breast cancer. It doesn't take an astrophysicist to see the benefit of adding an ultrasound to the screening process.

Yet for some years I've dealt with controversy over whether ultrasound adds benefit—or merely needless anxiety and cost.

In my practice we use two basic types of ultrasound, the standard diagnostic ultrasound and the whole breast screening ultrasound, and it's essential to understand the difference.

DIAGNOSTIC ULTRASOUND VERSUS WHOLE BREAST SCREENING ULTRASOUND— WHAT'S THE DIFFERENCE?

The standard diagnostic ultrasound has been around for decades. It's an important tool in evaluating breast lumps and is often used to distinguish abnormal changes on the mammogram. The ultrasound uses sound waves to bounce off breast tissue. It is completely painless. When a sound wave strikes an object, it bounces back or echoes. By measuring these echo waves, it is possible to determine the size, shape, and characteristics of a breast mass.

Whole breast screening ultrasound, however, is done in asymptomatic women whose breasts are found to be dense on the mammogram. The ultrasound exam evaluates the entirety of both breasts. This procedure differs from the diagnostic exam, which focuses on a specific area of concern, such as a lump or an abnormal spot on the mammogram. (It was the screening ultrasound that detected Joan Lunden's breast cancer that was missed on her screening mammogram—see page 102)

OTHER TYPES OF SCREENING TECHNOLOGIES: MRI AND 3-D MAMMOGRAPHY

It is well established that the MRI is the gold standard when it comes to early detection of breast cancers. The MRI relies on magnetic fields as opposed to X-rays (used for mammograms) or sound waves (associated with ultrasound technology) to create an image of the breast. It is performed with the patient in a tube, much like a CT scan. For this screening, a contrast material is injected into the patient's I.V. Cancer typically shows up with white density against a black background or in red, yellow, or blue, depending on the growth rate of the cancer.

The major drawback is cost—and because of this, insurance companies do not routinely cover it. The exception is that they will pay for high-risk women such as those with a strong family history of breast cancer. The out-of-pocket expense can be in the thousands of dollars, making it an impractical alternative for women who are at average risk for breast cancer.

Another bright spot on the horizon is tomosynthesis, or 3-D mammography. As opposed to the standard mammogram, which produces a two-dimensional image of the breast, this new technique creates a 3-D image, which gives the radiologist more detail, especially when looking at dense breasts. Studies show that the 3-D mammogram picks up more small cancers than the standard mammogram, and fewer patients are called back for additional mammographic views.

The 3-D mammogram is relatively new. The early models were associated with an increased dose in radiation, but newer models have mostly solved this problem. The 3-D mammogram is typically more expensive than the 2-D model.

One important, unanswered question is whether the 3-D mammogram can eliminate the need for ultrasound screening in women with dense breasts. We do see cases in which a cancer has been missed on the 3-D mammogram, but was seen on the screening ultrasound, so I still advise my patients with dense breasts to have ultrasound screening, even if their 3-D mammogram was normal.

Now that we are certain screening ultrasound works, the following questions need to be answered: First, just how good is it? Second, who needs it? And third, how often should it be done?

Should all women with dense breasts be advised to have one, or should it be limited to those women who successfully badger their insurance companies into paying for extra, and possibly unneeded, screening?

From my perspective, a 2012 study published in *The Journal of the American Medical Association (JAMA)* answered most of these questions. The study involved a total of 2,662 women with dense breasts who underwent yearly screening with both mammograms and ultrasounds.

The study was done over a period of three years. In that time, 110 new cancers were detected.

The take-home message from this study is that 32, or approximately one-third, of the cancers were seen only on the ultrasound. Thus, if not for the added screening, the diagnosis would have been delayed for most, if not all, of these 32 women.

I find this a startling conclusion—that approximately one-third of small cancers are missed on the screening mammogram. Stated another way, twice as many small cancers are detected when ultrasound screening is added to the traditional mammogram.

Critics point out that other studies have not found the screening ultrasound as effective as did the *JAMA* study. However, I am convinced that the *JAMA* experience set a new standard for such screening, and as technology improves, the ability to detect even more cancers missed on mammogram will get even better.

We have implemented an ultrasound screening program in our own practice, and, though the number of women involved is just over 1,000, its initial results are similar to those of the *JAMA* study. We are now detecting small cancers that have a high probability for cure but could have been killer cancers had they not been found on this additional screening. Our experience convinces me that other imaging centers can achieve similar results.

OUR CURRENT QUEST is to get the word out on this exciting new technology. For years I've been on a campaign to do just that, but until recently it's been an unending crusade. In my opinion, the medical community has been remiss in not promoting ultrasound screening. Their argument is seen all too frequently in medicine: The added cost does not justify the recommendation.

It's taken the actions of women such as Joan Lunden and Nancy Cappello to help spread the word that mammograms can miss cancers, and that, for women with dense breasts, ultrasound mammograms should be standard in the screening process.

A WOMAN WHO EXEMPLIFIES THE NEED
FOR EXTRA SCREENING

Joan Lunden, the former co-host of *Good Morning America*, is a TV icon who is well-known for her captivating smile and her beautiful blonde hair. In September 2014, she appeared on the cover of *People Magazine* with her winning smile, but absent the hair. Joan chose to appear bald to make a statement—to startle the public into an awareness of how mammograms can miss cancers.

The accompanying article explained that Joan was faithful in doing yearly mammograms, starting at age forty. Joan's most recent mammogram had been normal, but it showed her breasts were dense (as opposed to breasts that are termed "fatty"). Because of this, Joan's doctor suggested she have a whole breast screening ultrasound. A small lump was seen on the ultrasound, and a biopsy was recommended. The biopsy was positive for invasive breast cancer. Her cancer was small but also aggressive.

It is quite likely that the screening ultrasound saved her life.

Joan was lucky that her cancer was detected while still in an early stage. She owes her good fortune to another woman, who was not so lucky: Nancy Cappello.

ONE WOMAN'S FIGHT FOR CHANGE IN LEGISLATURE

Nancy Cappello was diligent about getting her yearly mammogram. Two months after receiving a normal screening mammogram, she found a ridge in her breast. A repeat mammogram was still normal, but a diagnostic ultrasound showed a suspicious mass. Her biopsy was positive. At surgery she was found to have a large cancer and thirteen positive lymph nodes.

Nancy was stunned. "How could this happen to me?" she asked her doctors. After all, she had done everything they told her to do, but she still ended up with advanced cancer. Nancy was not impressed with their answers. She was told it was routine not to inform women about their density status, because at the time no additional screening options existed as part of the diagnostic routine.

Nancy was smart enough to realize immediately that her doctors were missing the obvious. The solution for women with dense breasts was simply to add ultrasound to the screening process.

What she accomplished in the next few years was truly amazing. She took her story to legislators, and, in 2009, Connecticut became the first state to require that the ordering physician explain to women with dense breasts that mammograms have limitations and that other screening options, including ultrasound and MRI, must be considered. At the same time, insurance companies were required to cover ultrasound scans for these women. Nancy's home state, New York, followed soon after. Both have adopted legislation in favor of additional screening.

It would seem logical to assume that, once the new density status legislation (outlined in Nancy's story) passed, the problem was solved. Unfortunately, that has not been the case—the vast majority of women with dense breasts are still not aware of the potential lifesaving benefits of that second step, a screening ultrasound—and multiple barriers still must be surmounted.

Cost remains the biggest barrier. In many states, such as California, the law requires physicians to review screening options with their patients, but does *not* require insurance companies to pay. The out-of-pocket cost for an ultrasound in California ranges from $200 to more than $700. However, cost is only part of the problem.

In Connecticut, for example, the law requires insurance companies to pay for additional screening, and yet only a fraction of women are taking advantage of this new technology. Why?

In my experience, the answer to that question is not because of the cost. When I take the time to explain the pros and cons of additional imaging, most women conclude it is worth it. One patient pointed out,

"For the cost of a Diet Coke a day for a year, I could either save my life or be reassured my mammogram did not miss a breast cancer." I could not have said it better.

I am convinced two major reasons explain why women with dense breasts are not taking advantage of additional screening options: Either they have not been adequately informed by their physicians, or they are confused by mixed messages coming from the medical community.

Rather than focusing on the benefits of ultrasounds, some physicians and most insurance companies too often concentrate on the downside. They point out that ultrasound screening will lead to more biopsies and that some of these biopsies will prove *not* to be cancer. Thus, the message they send to women is that there will be added cost and anxiety, but with no medical benefits.

While they are correct in pointing this out, such a stance creates additional confusion. What women need is a balanced discussion of the pros and cons associated with ultrasound screening. Patients can then make an informed decision on what is in their best interest.

While I am fully aware of the problems associated with adding ultrasounds for the 50 percent of all women who are found to have dense breasts on mammograms, I am convinced that the benefits far outweigh the risks and costs. Joan and Nancy's stories, as well as those of hundreds of women from my own practice, have convinced me of the lifesaving value of ultrasounds. It's all too common for me to see patients for their second opinion who present large cancers that were missed on a prior mammogram but potentially could have been diagnosed much earlier with ultrasound.

SO, WHAT SHOULD a woman do if she is told her breasts are dense? Many states do not have legislation that requires doctors to discuss screening options with patients. In the states without such laws, most doctors do not have time to discuss all the imaging options with their patients.

Thus, the decision is left to the patient. In the absence of encouragement from physicians, the reality is all too clear: The majority of patients will not get the additional imaging they need.

My hope is that this book will inspire more proactive women such as Joan and Nancy to spread the word that mammograms are not the whole answer . . . that for certain women, additional ultrasound screening is not just optional—it saves lives!

WHAT I'D TELL MY DAUGHTER

- Average-risk women with dense breasts should consider having a yearly screening breast ultrasound in addition to their yearly mammogram.
- High-risk women (see Appendix I) should consider having a yearly MRI.

CHAPTER FIFTEEN

Shame on You, Dr. Krauthammer: Why He's Wrong About Mammograms

I REMEMBER TURNING on Fox News back in 2014 just in time to hear Bill O'Reilly announce on *The O'Reilly Factor*, his nightly television news program, that his next guest would comment on the controversy over the value of screening mammograms. The guest was none other than Dr. Charles Krauthammer. I was excited, not only because I believe Krauthammer is one of television's most brilliant commentators, but, more importantly, because he is also a fellow physician. I was confident he would get it right.

How wrong I was.

Dr. Krauthammer jumped right in with a shocking statement, asserting that a newly released Canadian study had proved that mammograms *do not save lives*. He praised the design of the research, which included 90,000 women who were followed over a period of twenty-five years. Half the group received regular mammograms, and the other half did not.

Then Dr. Krauthammer added that 20 percent of the women who were given a yearly mammogram were over-treated, meaning that they received unnecessary surgery, radiation, or chemotherapy. His conclusion implied that 20 percent of breast cancers detected on mammograms would have disappeared spontaneously without treatment. This bizarre conclusion was based on the observation that at the end of the investigation there was an equal number of deaths in both groups, but there were more breast cancers detected in the mammography group than in the group not receiving them. Another explanation for this seemingly inexplicable conclusion is that the study was flawed.

To me, the concept of breast cancers simply "disappearing" is one of the most outrageous conclusions in the history of medicine. There has never been a well-documented case of a single breast cancer vanishing without treatment. Yes, there are documented cases of breast cancers remaining stable over several years, but if followed long enough, most will eventually convert to a pattern of rapid growth.

The real reason there were more cancers in the mammography group is that more women who already had an existing breast cancer were placed there. From the start, the "randomization" that Dr. Krauthammer touted so highly was in fact not true. Because all the participating women were examined by nurses before being randomized, the nurses knew in advance which women had suspicious lumps, and which didn't. They also knew that the mammography group had been promised that they'd be treated in a timely manner, while those in the other group would receive the "usual care in the community." The nurses had an ethical dilemma. How could they allow a patient with an obvious cancer to be placed in a group in which treatment would be delayed? Thus, of the twenty-four women with large, locally advanced breast cancers, nineteen were assigned to the group getting mammograms. If these patients had been properly randomized, approximately twelve would be placed in each group. What actually happened was that, in some cases, women with obvious cancers were given the option of switching groups in order to get a timely mammogram and thus avoid treatment delays.

It was this basic flaw in the process of randomization that caused one of the early architects of the study, Dr. Norman F. Boyd, to go public with his concerns. He and his colleagues published a study in the journal *Radiology* criticizing the design of the study. Their report ends by saying, ". . . the results of these trials should not be used to change the prevailing scientific view of the potential benefits of screening with mammography." A polite way of stating the study's conclusions could not be trusted.

After listening to Dr. Krauthammer's assertion that mammograms not only don't work but also may cause harm, I was devastated. Dr. Krauthammer had accepted the conclusions of the Canadian study without the slightest reservations; worse, he'd implied that some dozen previous studies showing the lifesaving value of screening mammograms had now been proven wrong.

Because I assumed *The O'Reilly Factor* prided itself on being "fair and balanced," I expected the next guest to present the other side of the story. But there was no next guest. Apparently the opinion of Dr. Krauthammer was all the proof the show intended to offer.

IN RETROSPECT, it's not surprising that the Fox News story came out so lopsided. The fact that a large Canadian trial concluded that mammograms don't work is a hot topic. Everyone in the media wants to be the first to offer something startling—to trumpet Big News. This is the kind of juicy narrative that draws viewers and improves ratings. There was an urgency at Fox to rev up and get the story out, without a similar urgency to find a dissenting opinion. And having their own in-house physician with a high level of credibility (many viewers are so enamored with Dr. Krauthammer that his words are considered prophetic; to some fans, he is more than just a regular MD, he is an M.Diety) there was no need for Fox to search for someone opposed to their doctor's views.

Shortly after that appearance, the doctor was a guest on *The Kelly File*. To her credit, Megyn Kelly said that the subject of screening mammography was controversial and there was room for debate. She brought up Amy Robach's story as an example, attempting to bring some balance to the discussion.

A FAMOUS TV HOST DEMONSTRATES THE VALUE OF MAMMOGRAMS

Amy Robach, a co-anchor for *Good Morning America*, had recently turned forty, but had been putting off getting her first mammogram. Her co-anchor, Robin Roberts, who had previously been diagnosed with breast cancer, goaded Amy into undergoing her first screening. Amy relented, and to help get the word out on the importance of starting the procedure at age forty, she decided to be screened while doing her morning show.

She was stunned when she received a call a few days later indicating she had a suspicious spot on her mammogram. Shortly thereafter, a biopsy was performed and the spot proved to be an invasive breast cancer.

Megyn's attempt to air both sides of the discussion was ignored. Krauthammer remained adamant about the validity of the Canadian study, and again went on to praise its many virtues. He also repeated his assertion that 20 percent of patients in the mammography group received unnecessary treatment, including surgery and chemotherapy.

Following this second interview I went into a state of depression. In the past decade we had made incredible progress in detecting potentially curable breast cancers with improved screening techniques. I had been so optimistic about the future. It now appeared that all the momentum for better breast cancer care was coming to an end. I knew in my heart that if mammography guidelines were to be watered down, women, especially younger women, would die needlessly of advanced breast cancer.

AFTER THE TWO REPORTS from Fox News, it appeared that the media was reaching the consensus that screening mammograms did not work. The defenders of screening were almost completely ignored. The situation was becoming increasingly bleak for proponents of screening. But just when it seemed we were about to lose the battle, a new report came out of Canada.

This second investigation avoided the major flaws associated with the first. Breast exams were not performed on patients prior to entry, so the issue of bias was eliminated. As opposed to the original research, which used outdated equipment and poorly trained technicians, the second investigation employed state-of-the-art equipment. This time the technicians were well trained and the physicians received specific instructions in mammographic interpretation.

The results of the second investigation were made public in July 2014, six months after the findings from the first Canadian study were released. Overall, the project demonstrated a *40 percent reduction in breast cancer mortality*. It concluded, "Age at entry into screening did not greatly affect the average reduction in mortality." Thus, we now have clarity. Starting screening at age forty has the potential to reduce breast cancer deaths by up to 40 percent and could easily exceed 50 percent by adding additional screening with ultrasound and MRI for women with dense breasts.

In comparing the results of the two Canadian projects, the explanation for the failure of the first to show benefit was based on its inherent flaws. It takes a well-designed investigation with high-quality breast imaging to prove the effectiveness of mammographic screening. When studies are poorly designed and include outdated equipment and technicians with substandard training and scant experience, the diagnosis of breast cancer is delayed and mortality is increased.

The one indisputable conclusion to be made after reviewing the results of the initial Canadian project is that poor-quality mammography is bad for a woman's health. Although the initial Canadian investigation received worldwide media attention, not a peep was heard from the media about the results of the second. I would have expected some kind of response from *The O'Reilly Factor*, a validation of its claim to be "fair and balanced." This never happened.

CHAPTER SIXTEEN

❧

Mammograms:
The Spin Stops Here

D R. KRAUTHAMMER ISN'T THE ONLY ONE contributing to the
public confusion about mammograms, as we'll see. And that confusion has serious consequences, as it has already begun to lead to fewer
women in their forties getting mammograms.

Understanding the rationale for mammograms and their potential
to cut breast cancer mortality in half starts with understanding the
contributions of Dr. László Tabár, considered by his peers to be "the
father of mammography." How Dr. Tabár became a legend in his own
time is a remarkable story of one man's astonishing impact on women's
health. Dr. Tabár went to medical school in Hungary and received his
MD in 1967, the same year I received mine.

Early in his professional career, Tabár became fascinated with a
study from the United States that showed the benefit of mammographic
screening. The project was the first of its kind, commonly referred to as
the HIP study, for the Health Insurance Plan of Greater New York. It
followed two large groups of women for eighteen years. One group had
yearly mammograms and the other was not screened. Overall, there was
an approximate 30 percent reduction in breast cancer mortality in the

screened women—but it only benefited women fifty years and older. There was no survival advantage for women screened in their forties.

Dr. Tabár became intrigued with these findings. His instincts told him that the reason mammograms did not work for younger patients was because women in this age group tend to have dense breast tissue, which makes cancer detection difficult on mammograms. As women go into menopause, estrogen levels drop and density often decreases or disappears, making it easier to detect small cancers.

As explained in chapter fourteen, dense breast tissue appears white on the mammogram—but small cancers also show up as white spots (the snowman in a snowstorm). This problem sometimes makes it impossible to see even large cancers in women with dense breasts.

Tabár became obsessed with developing techniques for ferreting out the elusive white spots.

After graduating from medical school, he went on to get his PhD at the Hungarian Academy of Sciences, where his area of interest was breast cancer research, with a special focus on improving breast imaging quality. Dr. Tabár's timing could not have been better. Shortly after he received his PhD, a research position became available—for him, an opportunity almost too good to be true.

As it turned out, informed women in Sweden were excited about the lifesaving results from the American HIP study. A vocal group petitioned the government to establish a screening program in their own country. Sweden had a single-payer health care system and, like most health care entities, the Swedish health care system had a limited budget. If screening was introduced, it would need to be available to all Swedish women—and this would take a big bite out of money allocated for health care.

Before making such a major monetary commitment, the Swedish government wanted proof of benefit. They needed to find someone capable of accurately determining the value of mammographic screening and, after a worldwide search, they found that someone who had the background and motivation to take on such a project: Dr. Tabár.

Although he did not speak Swedish at the time, he was a quick learner. He assembled a team of prestigious research scientists, and together they produced a well-designed study to evaluate the potential benefit of mammography. Fortunately, Dr. Tabár was able to convince the government to include women in their forties, despite the lack of benefit previously noted in the HIP study.

Tabár was convinced that with refinements in technique, he could prove mammography's ability to reduce breast cancer mortality in all women—even those who were younger. In his quest to "find the snowman" in women with dense breasts, he developed new methods for doing a proper mammogram, mastered ways to process the films (which were not digital in those days), and learned how to detect the elusive anomaly in the mammograms of younger, dense-breasted women.

After three decades of study, the results were made public in 2011. Overall, breast cancer mortality in Sweden was reduced by almost 40 percent, and the mortality reduction for women in their forties approached 30 percent. This study remains the largest of its kind, with a longer follow-up than any other in the world.

IT SEEMS LOGICAL TO ASSUME that the Swedish study settled the controversy about starting screening at age forty. Once this issue was settled, the next goal should have focused on improving the quality of mammographic imaging, developing new technology, and lowering imaging costs.

Yet the controversy about the value of mammographic screening for younger women rages on. In fact, in the spring of 2015, the USPSTF (United States Preventive Services Task Force), a group sponsored by the U.S. government, concluded that screening women in their forties could do more harm than good. Shortly after the recommendations from the USPSTF were released, the American Cancer Society released a modification of their guidelines, recommending that average-risk women start yearly mammographic screening at age forty-five. Starting earlier, they said, should be based on a discussion of risk and benefits with a doctor.

I believe that the USPSTF put too much weight on the first badly flawed Canadian study (see chapter fifteen) to justify their recommendation to start screening at age fifty. Furthermore, it appears they ignored the second well-designed Canadian study that demonstrated a major reduction in breast cancer mortality for women who start yearly screening at age forty.

My conclusion is that this government-appointed committee had a mandate to put the brakes on spiraling health care costs, and thus had an inherent bias to cut spending. Of note, the only medical representation on the committee was from primary care physicians. There was no representation from experienced specialists (radiologists, surgeons, oncologists) who have firsthand knowledge of the value of starting screening at age forty. Thus the committee was able to pass recommendations that were based more on economics than on what is in the best interest of women in their forties.

The committee did admit, however, to a small reduction in breast cancer mortality associated with screening women in their forties. But their overall conclusion was both false and dangerous: A woman's anxiety, they claimed, associated with a negative biopsy due to an abnormal mammogram outweighed the benefits of screening.

The committee failed to note the emotional toll in a woman who learns a breast cancer diagnosis was delayed because she hadn't received appropriate screening. Nobody asked, "How could losing a few nights' sleep compare to receiving the news that your screening should have been done earlier, and now you need chemotherapy and your prognosis is uncertain?"

Instead, the committee recommended that screening start at age fifty and be continued every other year until age seventy-four, when screening should stop.

These are not just idle conclusions. Despite its lack of breast care specialists, the committee has unwarranted clout. Policy-makers in the government rely on the committee's "evidence-based" decision to set health care policy. Private insurance gatekeepers typically make policy decisions in concert with standards set by the government. Translated, this means the committee's recommendations provide insurance companies with an excuse for not covering mammography for women in their forties. It's also a cost-cutting alibi for such companies to pay only every other year for women fifty and older—and to stop funding mammograms entirely for women over age seventy-four.

There is no doubt in my mind that the committee's conclusions were strongly biased. The fact that they placed so much weight on the faulty Canadian study speaks for itself.

The reasons for these biases are obvious. Every year medical costs go up, until it appears they are literally spiraling out of control. Baby boomers are now signing up for Medicare, while expensive medical technologies continue to expand at an ever-increasing rate. Meanwhile, the public has an unquenchable thirst for expensive, cutting-edge services.

There are no easy solutions for this evolving crisis in health care, as demand increases and our ability to pay speeds in the opposite direction. It seems the only issue on which everyone agrees is the urgent need to put on the brakes for medical spending.

The question is, how do we address the problem of containing health care costs? It appears the federal government is now in panic mode. Congress desperately needs solutions to rising medical expenses, but cutting corners on breast cancer detection spells trouble. Costs of treatment will increase and benefits of early detection will diminish. Yet breast cancers will not go away. If not caught early, such malignancies will, in most cases, be detected as large lumps, as was the case in the era before organized screening.

The lifetime cost of treating an early-stage breast cancer is in the range of $50,000, and the probability for long-term survival is high. However, the lifetime cost of treating an advanced breast cancer can easily exceed $1 million, while the probability for long-term survival is markedly lowered. This calculation does not take into account loss of productivity or, more importantly, the loss of life. Nor are we considering that many deaths involve young mothers (also sisters and daughters), with the consequent devastation that death causes their families.

The government's approach to solving a complex medical issue with a task force of individuals who lack experience in the field they're regulating presents a clear example of how *not* to achieve better care or contain medical costs.

And yet solutions are available. Any medical researcher can find examples of other health care obstacles that were hurdled with a number of intelligent steps.

WHAT I'D TELL MY DAUGHTER

- Start screening mammograms at age forty, or earlier if you are high risk.
- Continue yearly as long as you are in good health.

CHAPTER SEVENTEEN

Your Bra: A No-Phone Zone

IFIRST BECAME AWARE of a potential relationship between breast cancer and cell phones in 2010, when I saw a patient of mine whom I'll call Sarah. Sarah was in her late thirties when she found a lump. A needle biopsy proved her lump was an invasive cancer. No one in her family had ever had this malady, and she was convinced her cell phone was the cause.

It is routine for us to present all newly diagnosed breast cancers to our weekly tumor board. In Sarah's case, she was presented to the board a second time because of the unusual findings on her recent pathology report on her mastectomy specimen. Rather than seeing a single focus of invasive growth, the pathologist had observed multiple areas of invasion covering a wide area of the specimen. The pathologist's description made me wonder if it was possible that Sarah was right.

At first, I kept my concerns to myself, since the possibility of a relationship between phone and tumor seemed to be such a long shot. Still, I found it hard to avoid thinking about the potential ramifications if such a link existed. I decided to present the case to a much larger group of breast care specialists.

A few months later, approximately sixty physicians, all of whom specialized in some aspect of breast cancer, attended a multi-specialty conference on new concepts in breast care. I summarized the case history, which included a description of the microscopic findings.

I was taken aback by their reaction. Rather than opening a debate, the group responded in unison, concluding there was absolutely no way a cell phone could cause breast cancer. The doctors were unanimous in agreeing that the relationship between the malignancy and the phone was coincidental. The group pointed out that millions of young women are exposed to cell phones. In this case, they said, it was just a coincidence that the cancer developed in the same area where the patient stored her device.

Over the next few years, several similar cases came to my attention; I was seeing more and more women who were convinced a cell phone caused their malignancy. By then I had adopted the party line, explaining there was no evidence that cell phones produce breast cancer. And yet, still other cases came to my attention.

THE PATIENT WITH THE ODD-SHAPED MALIGNANCY

A twenty-one-year-old woman, Jen (not her real name), was referred to our center because she noticed a bloody discharge coming from one of her nipples. The finding on her mammogram set up a firestorm of activity from our imaging department. I distinctly remember a group of technicians bursting into my office announcing, "We found another one!"

The mammogram was indeed unusual. It showed extensive malignant-appearing calcifications that seemed to have an odd rectangular distribution. I remember asking the radiologist, "What is the length and width of the calcifications?" She estimated it to be about 4½ inches by 2 inches. I asked her to measure the length and width of my cell phone. The match was nearly perfect. I was stunned.

It was Jen's case that convinced me that I needed to rethink the cell phone issue. However, though the findings on Jen's mammogram were impressive, they did not provide enough ammunition to convince me to go public. The memory of the negative reactions from my colleagues still burned in my mind. Before making my case, I needed a more convincing argument to support my claims.

Shortly after reviewing Jen's case, I did a second-opinion consultation on another young woman, recently treated for her breast cancer.

A PATIENT PROVES HER POINT

Rachel had what appeared to be a typical breast cancer. She had already undergone a lumpectomy and recently finished a six-week course of radiation therapy. She told me about an event that occurred during her first visit to the radiation department. In preparing her for treatment, a technician used a felt pen to outline the area to receive an extra dose of radiation.

She asked the technician, "Why the drawing?" The response was, "This is where your original cancer was located." Rachel looked at the drawing and lights exploded in her head. The drawing was in the shape of a rectangle. She reached for her cell phone (an old-fashioned flip phone) and placed it over the marking on her breast. It was an almost perfect match.

Looking back on her experience, Rachel wrote the following on Facebook: "I'm not an expert, nor a doctor, but I am one strong and determined woman with a whole lot of common sense. What I do know about breast cancer is that it doesn't grow four right angles that form a box that happens to be the same size as my cell phone. I have no doubt my cell phone was the cause of my breast cancer."

Rachel's case proved to be the final convincer. By then I felt a moral duty to make my concerns public. But I was also painfully aware that the medical community would remain skeptical, absent any scientific data to prove my point. Without convincing evidence, my theory would go nowhere.

I shared my reservations with Rachel, who was already well aware of the negative response from other physicians. She had spent a great deal of time trying to convince her doctors that cell phones could be dangerous. To her chagrin, her concerns were mainly ignored.

Now on a mission to get the word out, Rachel wanted my help. She explained to me that she had already done an extensive review of the safety guidelines in the cell phone manuals. She pointed out that seven years ago when she purchased her device, the user's manual, complete with safety guidelines, was included in the box with her new product. She clearly remembers reviewing the safety guidelines, which stated unequivocally that skin contact was safe.

Rachel pointed out two changes that have taken place since she purchased her original phone. First, she noted the manuals are no longer included with the appliance. The user is advised to go to the web for information. When she did a web search to review the manuals of the major cell phone manufacturers, she was stunned to find a reversal of their safety precautions. Buried in the middle of a 100-plus-page document, written in small print, was a section labeled "cell phone safety guidelines." Every manual she reviewed had the same advice: Avoid skin contact. The message couldn't have been clearer. But one manual went a step further. The BlackBerry manual also stated the following: "Failure to follow our safety guidelines could result in serious harm."

Rachel wondered what they knew that they were not telling the public. She also pointed out that government-sponsored safety guidelines were woefully out of date and completely ignored the issue of skin contact. In fact, the FCC did set safety standards for cell phone manufacturers. The guidelines, published in 1997, were designed to test the acute thermal effects, not to protect the consumer from radiation emitted from cell phones.

All this was useful information, but it was still not enough to convince a skeptical medical community. I needed to make a more compelling case if I wanted their support. Consequently, the next step was to review the scientific literature for clues that might support my suspicions. Unfortunately, the research to date is inconclusive, though the majority of researchers feel that more study is needed to obtain a definitive answer.

Yet there was one area of research that did convince me that a cell phone could do more than just warm up the skin, as my critics believed. Studies from infertility clinics have demonstrated a direct relationship between cell phone exposure and sperm counts. Not only were sperm counts low in the males who stored their cell phones in their front pockets, the sperm was abnormal in shape and did not move around normally. One month after the phone was removed, sperm counts and function returned to normal. This observation debunks the assertion by many scientists that the microwave energy emitted from such phones is too weak to have any negative impact on human cells.

Much of the reviewed information did support the concept that cell phones could cause breast cancer—but where was the proof? It finally dawned on me that we are unlikely to get that proof in my lifetime. The reality is that it takes decades to accumulate a sufficient number of cases to prove the issue one way or the other, as was the case with smoking and lung cancer. Decades prior to proving a direct relationship between tobacco use and malignancy in the lungs, many physicians were concerned that such a relationship did, in fact, exist. Yet skeptics continued to point to a lack of proof and suggested the relationship was just coincidental. After all, during the same time period, the rate of sugar consumption was also increasing. Yet no one except a comedian would suggest that sugar could cause lung cancer.

It took three decades to accumulate sufficient data to prove a direct relationship between the amount of tobacco consumed and the risk of developing lung cancer. It could easily take this long to get a final answer on the cell phone controversy. Yet, if there is such a risk, how will we explain to future generations our failure to be proactive?

Similarly, it took years to prove that chest X-rays could cause breast cancer. For decades, teenage girls with curvature of the spine (scoliosis) received chest X-rays with reckless abandon. It took thirty years to accumulate sufficient data to prove that these girls' developing breasts were highly vulnerable to radiation exposure. In short, what is perfectly safe for adult women could prove risky for teenage girls.

While thinking about the issue of chest X-rays causing breast cancer in teenagers, I had a eureka moment. Until now I had been going down the wrong path. Rather than trying to convince the medical community that cell phones could cause cancer, I needed an entirely different approach.

I decided to go public with a simple message. Rather than getting bogged down in a debate as to whether or not cell phones could cause breast cancer, I would focus on my personal experiences with young women who were diagnosed with phone-related breast cancers. I would admit that as yet we have no proof that cell phones can cause tumors, but my recent experiences suggest that such a link may well exist and that, since it may take decades to prove whether this risk is real, the prudent thing to do is to follow the manufacturers' advice and avoid skin contact.

Once secure in this new message, I was ready to hit the media. Within days, I was being quoted in newspapers, on television, and on the radio. It became a hot topic for bloggers—some of whom were very supportive, and others highly skeptical. Still, I was optimistic that all the hype would lead to demands from the public to take the issue seriously. After all, it was only two decades ago when a few ruptured silicone implants led to a major public outcry. Silicone implants were quickly removed from the marketplace. Women in need of reconstruction after breast surgery had to look for other less desirable options. Manufacturers went out of business and millions of dollars were lost.

How naïve I was: As quickly as the cell phone issue had become a hot topic, it disappeared from the radar. I didn't know what to do next. I had given it my best shot and failed.

Just when the subject indeed seemed dead, I learned about Tiffany Frantz: I received a call from Tracy, Tiffany's mother, who was also on a campaign to make the public aware of the cell phone issue. I was told that they were scheduled to be on *The Dr. Oz Show* in a couple of days. They invited me to be the medical expert. Realizing this was the break I was looking for, I immediately rescheduled my surgeries and took the red-eye to New York City.

TIFFANY CONVINCES DR. OZ

Twenty-three-year-old Tiffany looked angelic when she stood in front of a live audience and told Dr. Oz how a cell phone caused her breast cancer. Tiffany was candid about her personal tragedy—brave enough to share her private story with the world—but she had one secret she did not want to reveal to the audience—she had metastic cancer.

Tiffany's story started two years earlier when she found a lump in her breast. Not unduly worried at first, she became concerned when told she needed a biopsy. A few days later she received the report: At age twenty-one she was diagnosed with an invasive tumor. Two weeks after that she underwent a mastectomy with immediate reconstruction, and following surgery she was started on a course of chemotherapy.

Tiffany's mother, Tracy, explained to Dr. Oz how concerned she was when she first noticed that her then seventeen-year-old daughter was storing her cell phone in her bra. Tracy's intuition told her it was not safe, but she had no proof to back up her concerns. She tried to convince Tiffany to find some other receptacle, but, like many teenage girls, Tiffany dismissed her mother's advice.

Bonded to the device, Tiffany sent and received hundreds of text messages daily. Each morning she put the phone in her bra as she dressed, and only removed it at bedtime. Two years after Tiffany's diagnosis, she and her mother declared their campaign to make young women aware of the potential risk of developing a malignancy after a cell phone is placed in contact with their breasts.

The show was a great success. The audience fell in love with Tiffany as she shared her very personal story. As the show ended, Dr. Oz told me he was initially doubtful that cell phones could cause cancer, but after seeing the evidence he was convinced that it was a real issue. He stated that he would lead a campaign to make the bra a "No-Phone Zone." Fortunately, our conversation was being filmed, and that made a great ending to the interview.

As expected, there was an incredible media response. I received emails from many young women who were convinced a cell phone was the culprit in their own breast cancers. Yet shortly after my appearance on the show, one of my surgical colleagues wrote a scathing blog post describing Dr. Oz in the most unflattering terms. He also labeled me a charlatan and a fearmonger. Initially, I found the criticism upsetting. With time, I realized that such outbursts were inevitable, and I had to learn to deal with them. After all, bad publicity is better than no publicity.

DESPITE OVERWHELMING RESPONSE from the public and media, once again the topic soon faded from the limelight. The blogs went dead, and phone calls and emails dwindled to a trickle. Dr. Oz had provided me with the opportunity of a lifetime, but I had failed to capitalize on it. It was time for a new strategy, though I was at a loss for ideas to reinvigorate my campaign.

One approach that seemed promising was to investigate how other public health issues had been addressed. Since the connection between cell phones and breast cancer has similar elements to the proven link between smoking and lung cancer, I decided studying the tobacco saga might provide insights into new ways to alert women to possible dangers from their beloved phones.

While it is now an established fact that cigarette smoking is a direct cause of lung cancer, it took half a century to prove it. In the past, scientists were aware that rates of lung cancer were increasing at the same time that smoking was on the uptick. Many observers were convinced this was just a coincidence. In the late 1940s, one skeptical surgeon, when presented with this observation, noted that the use of nylon stockings was also becoming increasingly common.

In reviewing the tobacco question, I was surprised to learn that as early as the 1920s, scientific evidence suggested that tobacco use could produce serious malignancy. Yet it wasn't until the 1950s that British and American scientists established, once and for all, a direct link between smoking and diseased lungs.

Even then, it took the Surgeon General another twenty years to place warnings on cigarette packages. Finally, in 1999, the nation's largest supplier of cigarettes, Philip Morris, issued a statement admitting that cigarettes could cause lung cancer. I wondered why it took so long for the Surgeon General to step up. Or further, why Philip Morris 'fessed up at all.

The long delay in official action from the government was hard to understand—until you consider that the tobacco industry was politically powerful and a significant contributor to the American economy, both in terms of sales and a welcome source of tax revenue. Furthermore, in the 1950s, some quarter or more of Americans smoked.

But reasons for Philip Morris's owning up proved more subtle. In the end the corporation decided if they went public with the admission that smoking can cause lung cancer, they could provide a clear defense against future liability. In other words, if a smoker claimed that cigarettes caused his lung disease, Philip Morris could now argue that he had been warned.

Thinking about this, I realized cell phone manufacturers were doing the exact same thing by putting out subtle warnings to avoid skin contact. They were "covering" themselves, exactly as Philip Morris had done. They simply wanted to protect themselves from future litigation and subsequent liability. After all, if they were truly interested in protecting the public, they would have put their warnings in an obvious place, as the Surgeon General has finally done with cigarettes.

It's worth repeating that when the flip phone became available to the public in 1996, the safety manual was included in the box with the instrument. The original manuals implied that skin contact was perfectly safe. As Rachel discovered, manuals are no longer included with new phones. Instead they are posted on the internet, with safety guidelines buried in the middle of a long and complex document.

Lawyers for manufacturers knew what they were doing: Once this warning was made available, the cell phone companies would be protected against a claim that their product caused cancer. Their astute legal teams could argue that the public had been given sufficient warning about the risk of skin contact.

There is a final reason for suspecting manufacturers are manipulating the system. FCC guidelines for cell phone manufacturers are outdated. The FCC last put out such guidelines in 1997, which spoke to the amount of energy absorbed by an artificial head of a theoretical 200-pound male. The head was constructed of plastic and filled with a liquid that represents the electrical properties of human tissue, and the cell phone was placed a fraction of an inch from the head for a period of thirty minutes. The model could then measure the amount of radio frequency energy absorbed during the thirty-minute time period. This measurement is referred to as specific absorption rate, or, more commonly, SAR. The FCC then set an arbitrary threshold for SAR. Cell phone manufacturers are not allowed to sell phones that exceed this threshold.

It's obvious now that these guidelines do not adequately address basic health concerns. A thirty-minute time exposure is irrelevant to current usage. Our own study of college girls in our area, done by a pre-med student, showed some were storing their cell phones in their bras continuously for more than ten hours a day.

In the FCC report the question of skin contact was not addressed—nor was the matter of age at time of exposure. The topic of vulnerability of organs such as the brain or breast was also not considered. In short, the FCC guidelines are inadequate, arbitrary, and outdated.

When I think of how quickly the FDA responded to the silicone breast implant problem, I am at a loss to explain how another governmental agency, the FCC, can be so disconnected from what could be another major health matter. Is it possible they are being pressured by manufacturers? I have no direct evidence that this is the case. However, there is an urgent need for answers to basic questions. It is time for the public to demand them and time for the FCC to respond.

A FINAL COMPARISON between cigarettes and cell phones highlights the magnitude of today's concerns: Whereas a mere fourth to a third of Americans once smoked cigarettes, today nearly everyone has a cell phone.

However, there is good news: It's possible that things are about to change. In preparing for what could be the trial of the century (*Michael P. Murray vs. Motorola, Inc. et al*, in which a cell phone allegedly caused the plaintiff's brain cancer), Judge Frederick H. Weisberg offered the following statement:

> If there is even a reasonable possibility that cell phone radiation is carcinogenic, the time for action in the public health and regulatory sectors is upon us. Even though the financial and social cost of restricting such devices would be significant, those costs pale in comparison to the cost in human lives from doing nothing, only to discover thirty or forty years from now that the early signs were pointing in the right direction. If the probability of carcinogenicity is low, but the magnitude of the potential harm is high, good public policy dictates that the risk should not be ignored.

He spoke for all of us.

In response to growing public concern about cell phone safety, the NIH funded a $25 million study to be conducted by the National Toxicology Program (NTP) to help clarify the potential health hazards from exposure to cell phone radiation.

The initial results of their study have been released, and the result are strongly suggestive that cell phone exposure can cause cancer. The study found that one in twelve male rats exposed to cell phone radiation developed cancer or a pre-cancerous lesion as compared to no cancers in the group of rats that were not exposed to cell phone radiation.

These are preliminary findings, and the debate will undoubtedly intensify as further study results become available. Although there are many questions left to be answered, there is now convincing evidence that cell phones can cause cancer. It is time for skeptics to admit that the prudent approach for every woman is to make the bra a "no phone zone."

WHAT I'D TELL MY DAUGHTER

- Avoid skin contact with your cell phone.
- Keep your cell phone out of your bra.

CHAPTER EIGHTEEN

Genetic Testing

THE ANNOUNCEMENT CAME as a shock to her fans: Angelina Jolie was about to have both breasts removed. Considered one of the most beautiful women in the world, she took this momentous step to lower her risk of developing breast cancer. But her decision did more than alter her body—it forever transformed the future of genetic testing.

Every mother could understand Angelina Jolie's motivation for such a drastic measure. As a teenager, the actress had watched her mother's heartbreaking downhill course as she slowly succumbed to her battle against ovarian cancer. Angelina wanted to make certain her own children would not suffer the same fate, and she hoped to live long enough to hold her grandchildren in her arms.

Here is a classic example of a woman at high risk of developing breast cancer. Among her closest relatives were a number of women with both breast and ovarian cancers. Yet she was the first among them to be tested for a BRCA gene mutation—and she tested positive, meaning her risk of developing breast or ovarian cancer was greatly increased.

In March 2015, Angelina wrote an article for *The New York Times* explaining her rationale for having a double mastectomy. She noted in the text that her surgery lowered her lifetime risk of developing breast cancer from 87 percent to 5 percent. This was a remarkable improvement, considering that the average woman has a 12-percent lifetime risk of acquiring the disease.

Following her surgery, Angelina made it perfectly clear that she felt every bit as feminine as she did before the operation. She stated that her husband, Brad Pitt, was incredibly supportive, and, if anything, their relationship was even stronger afterward. In my experience, Angelina's sense of relief following her procedure is nearly universal among women who have had a similar risk reduction surgery.

WHAT'S IN YOUR GENES?
TESTING FOR BRCA MUTATIONS

Prior to Angelina's announcement, the issue of genetic testing was rarely discussed, even among women with family histories of breast cancer. In large part, this lack of public awareness was due to the fact that testing of the BRCA genes had only recently become available, and the cost of performing the test was prohibitive.

For decades, the medical community has been aware of families in which multiple generations of women have had both breast and ovarian cancers. In 1994, Dr. Mary-Claire King, who had been studying the genetics of these high-risk families, discovered the first gene that caused hereditary breast cancer. A few months later, in 1995, a second breast cancer gene was found. These two genes are referred to as BRCA1 and BRCA2. Everyone has both genes—they play a protective role in the body. But when there is a mutation in one of them, the protective function doesn't work as well, putting women at a much higher risk for breast and ovarian cancers.

Though both males and females can carry a mutation, the probability of men developing breast cancer is much lower than for women. If either parent carries a gene mutation, each child will have a fifty–fifty chance of inheriting it.

It took more than a decade from the discovery of the two BRCA genes to the development of a practical test to determine whether a particular woman was affected. At the time of Angelina's diagnosis, Myriad Genetics was the only company in the world that could run the test to determine whether someone was a mutated-gene carrier. Myriad had patents on these genes and thus controlled the test price. The out-of-pocket cost to the consumer could exceed $4,000. At first, insurance companies were reluctant to pay for the test, or they downright refused. For them, it was not just the one-time expense. The companies were concerned that eventually every woman might demand genetic testing, thus escalating the overall cost of care and potentially reducing their profits.

In an effort to put pressure on the insurance companies to cover at least part of the expense, physicians would typically send high-risk patients to genetic counselors. These experts would do a rigorous multigenerational family review. They were particularly interested in finding relatives who would be considered a "red flag" for the presence of a gene mutation.

Within a family, typical examples of "red flags" would be women under fifty afflicted with breast cancer, or women with cancers in both breasts. Others would include families with a history of ovarian cancers or male breast cancers, or those of Ashkenazi Jewish heritage, because women of this background are at high risk of carrying a BRCA mutation. While the chance of a mutation for the average woman is approximately one in four hundred, for women of Ashkenazi heritage (who, with European ancestry, make up the majority of American Jews) the figure changes to one in forty.

A MAN'S ROLE IN GENETIC MUTATIONS

A sixty-two-year-old man with an Ashkenazi background learned of the risk of mutation in women of his ethnic group. There was no history of breast or ovarian cancer in his family. He had three daughters, all in their late teens or early twenties. Despite the lack of family history, he decided to pay out of pocket to be tested for the gene. Much to the surprise of the skeptical genetic counselor, he tested positive. Now, all of his Jewish relatives, including his three daughters, are on notice. In essence, the odds of his closest relatives carrying the BRCA mutation have shifted from one in forty to fifty–fifty.

This father's story does not end with the positive BRCA test. The fact that he tested positive for the damaging gene puts him at increased risk for other cancers such as prostate and pancreatic. In fact, the man underwent extensive cancer screening and was found to have a small prostate cancer that, because of early screening, had an excellent prognosis. His proactive approach to cancer likely saved his life.

These high-risk populations, based primarily on their family histories, were—until recently—the only ones for whom insurance companies were required to pay for testing, which at that time was in the range of several thousand dollars—meaning insurance companies were rigid and stuck to strict criteria for who should be screened (see NCCN guidelines in Appendix I).

However, around the time of Angelina's diagnosis, revolutionary changes were taking place in the world of genetic testing. In the past two years the issue of identifying women at risk for a gene mutation has become ever more puzzling. For years we have sent women with very strong family histories to genetic counselors, only to find many did not carry a BRCA gene mutation. We supposed there must be other genes floating around that increased a woman's chance of developing the disease, but we could only guess about their presence, since they were yet to be discovered. Now we know that the doctors had it right.

In the past few years, research scientists have discovered at least thirty more high-risk genes that, when mutated, increase a woman's chance of developing breast and other related cancers. Now, rather than just testing women for the BRCA genes, we do "panel testing," which includes these other new genes. The number of new high-risk genes is expanding rapidly.

This discovery is only one of the major breakthroughs for genetic testing. For years there was ongoing debate about the legality of Myriad holding the patents on the BRCA genes. The Supreme Court ultimately solved the controversy in 2013. It ruled that no one could hold a patent on DNA. The court declared that this was a naturally occurring substance that was "owned" by the general public. Companies were allowed to hold patents on methods of *testing* DNA, but not on the DNA itself. The logjam was finally broken.

Almost overnight, multiple companies came on the scene and aggressively marketed their BRCA tests to any physician who would listen. As expected, competition led to price reductions, followed immediately by a rapid expansion in the number of women being tested.

A new company called Color Genomics offers comprehensive genetic testing for $249, which includes testing both BRCA genes (BRCA1 and BRCA2) and twenty-eight additional genes that are associated with an increased risk of developing breast and ovarian cancer. It helps that the company also provides financial assistance to women who cannot afford to pay. As a result, Color Genomics has greatly reduced cost as a barrier to genetic testing.

Another benefit offered by the new company is making their testing readily available to anyone who is interested. And further, women are no longer required to seek genetic counseling to determine whether they qualify. Women (and men) can now go directly to the Color Genomics website and review the educational videos. If they decide to participate, they need only pay $249 in advance and have their physician fax a signed order form, or an online physician can do this, and the report will be sent to the patient's doctor. Shortly after someone makes the payment, a test kit arrives. Patients follow the simple instructions and return the kit with a sample of their own saliva. Patients are also asked to provide information on their personal and family histories. Results are usually available in four to eight weeks (and that interval will get shorter in the near future). A team of genetic counselors is available to discuss the results with the patient and their physician.

This bold new approach to genetic testing will almost certainly turn the world of hereditary cancer screening upside down. It is too early to determine the magnitude of its impact, but this novel approach to testing has already generated a firestorm of criticism from experts who still support the established process of having genetic counselors see the woman first to determine whether she is a candidate. And it raises the question: Now that genetic testing is becoming widely available, should all women receive screening?

SHOULD EVERY WOMAN UNDERGO GENE TESTING?

Family history has always been the key factor in determining who needs this type of testing and who doesn't. But it is now becoming apparent that family history alone will miss a large number of women who are carriers. Most women who carry a BRCA mutation will have a family history of breast or ovarian cancer—but it is becoming increasingly clear that some women are at risk of carrying the gene, but are completely unaware of their high-risk status.

One obvious at-risk group is women who were adopted and don't know their family history. Another would be women who unknowingly carry a mutation from the male side of the family. Men with the mutation rarely get breast cancer, but there is a fifty–fifty chance they will pass the aberrant gene to each child.

A CLASSIC CASE OF A SILENT CARRIER

Our patient, Caitlin, was forty-two years old when she presented to our center with a large breast cancer. Because she had no family history of malignancy—either breast or ovarian—she underwent gene testing because of her young age. Her testing was routine, based on established guidelines (see Appendix I). Everyone was shocked when she tested positive for a BRCA gene mutation.

After an extensive search, it was discovered that her great-grandfather had been diagnosed with breast cancer. Until Caitlin's diagnosis, this ancestor's illness had remained a dark family secret. Detecting BRCA mutation in families where a male is the silent carrier is one of medicine's many challenges.

In retrospect, it became obvious that her great-grandfather must have had a BRCA mutation. He then passed it on to her grandfather, who in turn donated it to her father. Ultimately the father's gene went to Caitlin.

This concept of "silent carriers" of high-risk gene mutations comes as a great surprise to most women and a large number of physicians. Until recently, the issue was off our radar. I myself had never considered discussing the possibility of a high-risk mutation with women who did not have a family history of breast cancer until I read a lecture by Dr. King, the woman who first discovered the BRCA1 mutation and has championed the concept of testing all women by age thirty.

In 2014, Dr. King received the prestigious Lasker Award "for her bold and imaginative contributions to medical science and society . . . exemplified by her discovery of a single gene, BRCA1, that causes a virulent form of hereditary breast cancer." In her acceptance speech, she outlined her rationale for recommending all young women be given the opportunity for BRCA1/2 testing. She noted that the current restricted approach to screening for high-risk gene mutations fails to identify many women who are mutation carriers, though completely unaware of their risks. In her previous studies, Dr. King found a disturbing number of women who carried a mutation but had no family history of either breast or ovarian cancers.

In her lecture, she made the point that if we knew in advance that a woman was a "silent carrier" we could offer advice that could prove to be lifesaving. This almost certainly would have been the case with patients like Caitlin. For example, if Caitlin were identified as a BRCA mutation carrier at age thirty, as recommended by Dr. King, she could have been given the option of aggressive screening. As we've pointed out, we know that yearly MRI screening is highly effective in detecting small breast cancers in high-risk women with dense breasts (see chapter fourteen). In Caitlin's case, a yearly MRI would have led to an earlier diagnosis without the need for such aggressive treatment.

Alternatively, Caitlin could have opted to have both breasts removed with a prophylactic nipple-sparing mastectomy and immediate reconstruction (see chapter twenty-five). Had she done this, the overwhelming odds are that she would never have developed breast cancer in the first place.

Dr. King also made the important point that detecting genetic mutations in young women after a diagnosis of breast cancer becomes a "failure of prevention." The numbers speak for themselves. Approximately 230,000 new cases of invasive breast cancer are diagnosed yearly. It is estimated that 5 to 10 percent of these women will carry a high-risk gene mutation. With a painstaking approach to population screening, most of the "silent carriers" could theoretically be identified prior to developing a breast cancer. Thus, aggressive genetic screening has the potential of saving thousands of lives every year.

ONE FAMILY'S BATTLE WITH "OTHER" MUTATIONS

About twenty-five years ago, I received a call from a distraught family who told me their twenty-four-year-old daughter, Merle (her real name), had just been diagnosed with breast cancer. She was flying home from a college in the Midwest. To say the family was anxious to start treatment would be an understatement.

I first met Merle at her home on a Sunday morning. She had a lemon-sized mass in her left breast that was an obvious, very large breast cancer. Merle was remarkably composed, but the anxiety of her parents and her three sisters could not have been greater. "We so thank you for coming to our home on a Sunday," said the mother, and it was clear the family was greatly relieved to learn that Merle would receive immediate medical attention.

A few days later we started her on chemotherapy. Unfortunately, the tumor proved to be extremely aggressive. Back then we lacked the sophisticated chemotherapies that are now available to treat more aggressive cancers. Even while she was receiving chemo, the tumor continued to grow. Merle died before reaching the age of twenty-five.

It is rare for us to see breast cancer in women in their early twenties. We were suspicious that something unusual was going on, but we had no idea what it might be. When BRCA testing became available, we expected to get an answer, but to our surprise her mother and all three sisters tested negative. For a long time, I continued to follow the family.

Two years ago, panel testing became available, and I was anxious to see if it would provide an explanation for why Merle developed breast cancer at such an early age.

We first tested the three sisters, and two were positive for a newly identified gene mutation. To our astonishment, each sister had a different variant of the same gene. A likely explanation is that one girl received a mutation from one parent and her sibling inherited a different mutation from the other.

These facts may also explain Merle's very aggressive cancer. It seems likely she received both mutations (one from each parent), and the combination led to the development of an unusually aggressive cancer, which showed up at an early age.

ONGOING CONTROVERSIES:
LOW-COST GENETIC TESTING

Despite the potential benefits of widespread screening, many experts in the field of human genetics believe the concept is not ready for prime time. They contend there are many ambiguities about the nature of cancer-causing genes, and they believe it is premature to rush into a more vigorous approach before we've had more experience in testing women who meet standard guidelines—and thus are obviously at high risk for mutations.

The critics express concern that a more aggressive approach to screening could result in increased levels of anxiety in young women, the majority of whom will not be gene carriers. As one patient said to me, "I've noticed how often a woman's possible 'anxiety' is used as an excuse for medical inaction. Men seem to see us as wilting heroines in old-fashioned novels—swooning away, unable to endure the slightest hints of uneasiness."

An additional concern is that women who test negative for a genetic mutation will become complacent and not participate in recommended high-risk screening. Many women with strong family histories of breast and ovarian cancer test negative for a mutation, but are still considered to be at high risk for developing a future breast cancer and need aggressive long-term screening.

These women need careful follow-up, including yearly MRI screening. They also must understand the need for additional genetic testing in the future as new high-risk genetic mutations are identified.

Women who use the internet to obtain genetic testing may not be adequately informed about one of the current disadvantages of gene testing. Although health insurance companies are not allowed to deny coverage or charge higher premiums for women who test positive for a high-risk mutation, there is no similar protection from life insurance companies or disability insurance providers who might deny coverage.

Despite the potential problems of a web-based approach to gene testing, we have become strong advocates of the concept. However, we continue to use established genetic testing labs for ordering gene testing for women who meet the established criteria (see Appendix I). Insurance covers the cost of testing for most women who meet the criteria, and the out-of-pocket cost is often less than the price of a web-based alternative. Also, we can expect to obtain results in a shorter time frame, which is important for women who are newly diagnosed with breast cancer and are considering their surgical treatment options.

Once the Color Genomics model was introduced into the marketplace, it immediately became apparent to us that this approach was of major value to patients with strong family histories who did not quite qualify for gene testing by standard guidelines. Out-of-pocket costs that would have been several thousand dollars are now closer to $250.

A second group of patients who have benefited from low-cost testing are women who have previously been diagnosed with breast cancer—with little or no family history of breast or any other cancer. Despite their lack of family history, they remain concerned they could be "silent carriers." Here their concern is not so much for themselves, but for their children and grandchildren. We have found that most of our breast cancer patients jump at the chance to be tested at a reasonable cost.

CURRENT PRACTICE AT OUR CLINIC

At my clinic, we have yet to address the issue of encouraging testing of all women by the age of thirty. For patients who express an interest, we do provide literature on Color Genomics, but we have not yet established a policy to encourage all young women to be tested by age thirty, as recommended by Dr. King.

I assume many young women will be sufficiently concerned to review the options on the Color Genomics website. But are we prepared to accept Dr. King's challenge and promote the concept of population-based testing for all young women? That's the next big question.

I believe knowledge is power. Our current approach to genetic testing is not perfect, but as Dr. King noted in her recent lecture, waiting for the perfect test denies women the opportunity to take advantage of the excellent resources that are currently available. We are in the midst of a revolution in gene testing. It's a sea of change that will profoundly impact how we care for women at risk. With the cost of testing falling precipitously, there is now an urgent need to streamline our risk assessment program.

We have reached the point where every woman would benefit from an early and accurate assessment of her personal cancer risk. Each woman should have a personalized plan to identify her probabilities, a strategy for reducing those risks when possible, and a clear agenda for early detection.

However, there are simply not enough genetic counselors to meet this challenge, and we are in urgent need of a practical approach to make testing happen. One procedure that has revolutionized our practice is to train mid-level providers, such as nurse practitioners and physician assistants, to do risk screening on our patients. As it is, we only refer the very complicated cases to genetic counselors.

At our center, we do risk screening on all new patients who come to us, including those who just appear for screening mammograms and those who are there to see one of our breast care specialists. We have a risk assessment program that is designed for all women, whether they have a family history or not.

The program deals with all aspects of risk assessment, starting with a family history and including other well-defined risk factors, such as exposure to radiation at a young age. We even mention avoiding skin contact with cell phones. We discuss screening options for women with dense breasts, plus issues of lifestyle, such as exercise, diet, and alcohol intake, which are the three modifiable risk factors.

A major focus of the program is on family history, which is not a modifiable factor. Each patient is instructed to get as much information as possible on all cancers in the family. This information is then fed into a series of computer programs that give a specific measure of risk (see Appendix I). Such programs help decide who needs an MRI and who needs genetic testing. Patients are given a detailed assessment of their personal risks along with a plan of action that provides specific recommendations on how to address them.

Patients are encouraged to reassess risk on a yearly basis, and to re-calculate based on any new information on family history—or even on the availability of newly detected genes that might influence their personal hazards.

THE FUTURE OF GENETIC TESTING

The roller coaster ride on the genetic express has just begun. One exciting treatment breakthrough provides a glimpse of what might be in store eventually. Among the greatest fears of individuals who carry a BRCA mutation is that they will pass their mutation to the next generation. For families concerned about this possibility, it is now technically possible to test embryos before in-vitro fertilization. Embryos that carry the mutation can be discarded and only those with normal BRCA genes selected for implantation.

As we enter this brave new world of gene testing that may well include comprehensive genetic studies even prior to birth, there will be a predictable outcry from critics who suggest we are playing God. Routine testing at birth will have profound ethical dilemmas—as well as problems with privacy issues.

In considering these imponderables, it is important that we do not lose sight of the fact that progress in genetic testing has the potential for not only saving lives, but reducing the potential for pain and suffering.

WHAT I'D TELL MY DAUGHTER

- Learn as much as you can about your family history of cancer.
- Consider risk assessment counseling if you have a family history of breast or ovarian cancer.
- Carefully consider the pros and cons of genetic testing now that cost is no longer a major barrier.

SECTION V

Prevention

CHAPTER NINETEEN

Beating the Genetic Odds: Exercise, Diet, and Weight Control

O̲UR GENETIC CODE is set at the moment of conception, and we are basically stuck with whatever genetic risks we inherited from our parents. Although such risks are fixed, and may require extra—and earlier—screening, women are not limited to screening remedies. Important lifestyle changes can also have a major influence on a woman's probability of developing breast cancer.

EXERCISE

Heading this list of modifiable risk factors is exercise. I often tell my patients that the top three things you can do to improve your health and reduce your chance of developing breast cancer are: *exercise, exercise,* and *more exercise.*

Physical activity not only reduces a woman's likelihood of getting breast cancer, it protects against other significant health problems such as heart disease and diabetes. A further remarkable benefit of exercise is its calming effect. In fact, regular workouts have been shown to be just as effective in treating depression as a popular antidepressant.

In the not-so-distant past, physical exertion was a natural component of everyday life. You had to burn a lot of calories just to survive. Now we drive cars, take elevators, and sit for long hours in front of computers and television screens. Today, leading what is considered a "normal" life means we use only a fraction of the calories our ancestors expended on a daily basis.

When I ask my patients why they don't exercise, the most common answer is, "I just don't have time." Despite all the labor-saving devices at our fingertips, life has become so hectic for most of my patients that they are convinced they don't have minutes to spare for this one vital activity.

As it turns out, it doesn't take a lot of those minutes to get at least some of the important benefits of exertion. Recent studies have shown a woman can lower her chance of developing breast cancer by walking only thirty minutes a day for five days a week.

This daily exercise is something every woman should be able to fit into her busy schedule. It starts with a new, positive attitude. As the Nike ad states, "Just do it." Take the stairs instead of the elevator. Park your car away from your destination. Take a walk around the block on your lunch break. Make it fun; walk with friends.

With a little imagination, most women should be able to exercise the basic thirty minutes a day and still accomplish all their goals. In fact, I predict that the positive vibes you get from exercising will actually increase your productivity and make you feel better about life in general. Exercise is free. It's the best bang for the buck you can get when investing in your own personal health care.

DIET

A common question I get from patients is, "Why are so many young women getting breast cancer?" I am convinced that diet is one of the prime factors leading to an increase in early-age cancers, meaning women in their twenties and thirties. Just as we have become too busy to exercise, our lives have become too fragmented for us to eat properly.

Fast food, packaged foods, and processed foods are cheap and convenient. They are also seductively tasty. When given the choice between buying a loaf of white bread or baking (or buying) a loaf with natural ingredients, the decision for the vast majority of Americans is a no-brainer. In fact, the very thought of home baking would never occur to most younger Americans. Looking back, it is hard to imagine when even our grandmothers had the time to bake bread.

Carbohydrates

Mounting evidence suggests that our carbohydrates are killing us. The first step to a healthy diet is to understand how such seemingly innocent nutrients are at the heart of our obesity epidemic. Carbs are an important part of most diets, and the trick is to distinguish between the good ones—like whole grains, brown rice, beans, and chia seeds—and those that are bad. By bad carbs, I am not just referring to sugary products such as candies, cakes, and cookies. I point to the ones most common to our diet—those that have undergone extensive processing, such as the starch we get in breads made with white flour, and, yes, ever-present items such as pasta and noodles. Eating such products is basically the same as eating table sugar.

Understanding how good carbs are turned into bad ones provides insight into the obesity problem. In fact, today's refined white flour is a classic example of what has gone wrong with our diets.

Initially, flour came from ground-up wheat seeds. Our ancestors learned to grow wheat about 10,000 years ago, a discovery that provided a stable food supply—a source of nutrition that enabled the early development of cities. In those days, the wheat seed was converted to flour with a grinding process that was slow but effective. The seeds were placed on a stone floor and a stone wheel pulled by animals ground the seeds into powder, or whole-wheat flour. This stone-ground flour was highly nutritious but labor intensive.

About 200 years ago, a process called milling replaced the wheel, which accelerated the rate at which grain could be converted to flour. The milling process removed the outer layer of the wheat seed, making the resulting flour less nutritious, though the resulting flour was used for a type of bread that had a longer shelf life and, for some people, tasted better.

The obvious drawback of this milling process was that, along with other valuable nutrients that were now absent, an element known as fiber was largely eliminated. Understanding the role of fiber is essential to grasping how a good carb can be converted to a bad one. The explanation is simple: Fiber slows the absorption of calories that are contained in the seed.

With the fiber gone, the calories are absorbed immediately, about as fast as if you were actually eating sugar. The net result works in several negative ways: First, you get hungry much sooner. Second, thanks to this lack of fiber, the bad carbs are absorbed so rapidly that the body is overwhelmed. It can't burn the carbs fast enough, so the excess calories are "stored" as or converted to fat. Picture cellulite in your mind and you get the idea.

A final downside: With fiber-free calories quickly metabolized, the body puts out high levels of insulin to "fight back" and keep blood sugar levels under control. It is well-known that insulin is a "growth promoter," meaning that prolonged presence of insulin may stimulate breast tissue and lead to an increased risk of developing breast cancer.

So how do we escape this plethora of undesirable carbohydrates? The simplest way is to avoid packaged or processed foods, including anything in a box, a can, or a package. It is best to eat whole grains (barley, wheat berry, chia seeds), fruits (but leave the skins on, and forget juices), beans, and vegetables that are rich in nutrients, such as broccoli.

If you do buy packaged or processed foods, it's essential to study the nutrition labels, not just the statements on the front, which are often misleading. For example, the cereal Froot Loops is labeled a "smart choice" when in reality it contains mostly sugar and no fruit. It's the nutrition labels that tell us what we need to know. Carbohydrates are listed in the middle of the section called Nutrition Facts. Here, our focus should center on "grams of carbohydrate." Under "carbohydrates" are posted both fiber and sugar in grams. In the case of original Froot Loops, the package admits to 20 grams of carbohydrate and 1 gram of fiber. (Recently, more fiber has been added, but still it is not a very smart choice.) Translated, a 20:1 ratio is essentially the same as eating pure sugar.

A major key to purchasing the best carbohydrate-containing foods is to make sure the fiber content is high. For example, if you are looking for bread that is not pure sugar, try to find one with a 5:1 carb to fiber ratio, or better. If you locate a label that states 20 grams of carbohydrate and 4 grams of fiber or more . . . bingo, you've got it. Finding bread, cereal, and other packaged products that meet or exceed the 5:1 ratio is not difficult— big retailers such as Costco have many nutritious breads to choose from.

Fats

The take-home message is simple: Fats don't make you fat; it's the carbs that make you fat. Why? Fat is a high-energy food, but it is absorbed slowly and provides sustained energy. In other words, you burn off the calories from fat as long as you don't overdo them.

However, some should be avoided, such as trans and saturated fats. Trans fats are found in processed foods such as bacon and lunch meats. There is a well-established relationship between high trans-fat intake and cardiovascular disease. Although there is less data to support the belief that trans fats are associated with an increased risk of developing breast cancer, there is sufficient data for both conditions to support the recommendation for lowering trans-fat intake.

It is better to get your calories from plant fats like those found in olive oil and avocados. Substituting plant fat calories for those in animal fats and white-flour carbs is an important step in converting to a wholesome diet.

Protein

Protein is essential to healthy eating. But dieticians raise legitimate concerns about the saturated fats in such protein-rich foods as red meat. Chicken and fish are probably better choices for protein—at least most of the time.

But we shouldn't overlook the value of plant-based proteins, such as those found in beans, barley, and nuts, which, for many of us, are a reasonable way to augment our daily intake of this important nutrient.

Nuts

Finally, I'd like to note an important source of protein. For the past year I have routinely asked my patients to name the one food that is proven to help you live longer. The most common guess is broccoli.

My patients are surprised to learn the truth: The real answer is nuts. A thirty-year study of 118,962 people, reported in the November 2013 *New England Journal of Medicine,* demonstrated that people who ate nuts lived longer—and the more nuts they ate, the longer they lived. Not only did they live longer, but they were also less prone to heart disease and cancer. In general, they were healthier than individuals who did not eat nuts. Fortunately, subjects who consumed peanuts did just as well as those who ate mixed nuts.

Now for an additional surprise: People who ate the most nuts had the lowest average weights. How could this be? After all, nuts are full of fat. See the next section for an explanation that is surprising to most of my patients.

WEIGHT CONTROL

Obesity is an established risk factor for developing breast cancer. Getting the weight off and keeping it off is a major task for many of my patients. The first two steps to long-term success are exercise and thoughtful eating (avoiding those fiber-free carbs).

Over the years I've gathered a series of tips that work when it comes to shedding pounds. The following are my top eight suggestions to complement diet and exercise:

1. **Stop eating as soon as you feel full.** We have two voices in our brains that influence how much we eat. The first comes from our primitive brain, telling us to eat all we can because we may not get another meal soon. The second, today's voice, tells us to stop eating because overeating has adverse consequences. The trick is to listen to the voice that tells us we're full.

2. **Snack properly.** Again, one of the major reasons for "filling up" is the primitive concern that we won't eat enough to make it to the next meal. One of the important strategies to dieting, therefore, is to avoid going hungry. The hungrier you get, the more driven you become, and the more likely you are to make poor food choices and overeat.

   Thus, it's important to snack properly. Let's say, for example, you have a good breakfast but stop eating as soon as you start feeling full. Chances are, you'll be hungry before lunch. Two choices emerge: suffer through it (not a long-term solution), or snack properly. Here, a small bag of raw almonds at your fingertips can solve the problem—especially if eaten slowly, then discontinued when the hunger abates.

   As one of my patients told me, "I love nuts; they fill me up."

   I find pine nuts, which are actually seeds, to be another excellent choice. There is evidence that pine nuts contain a substance that suppresses the appetite, possibly making them the ideal snack for dieters.

There are plenty of other options. Instead of a smoothie, try this: For liquid supplements I dilute chia seeds in water and add fresh-squeezed lemons and pureed berries. It tastes great and has a very high fiber to carbohydrate ratio.

3. **After every meal, brush your teeth and gargle.** I am convinced that brushing and gargling after meals sends a message to the brain that the meal is over. In response, the brain stops sending messages to eat more.

4. **Start with small servings.** It is no longer a crime not to eat everything on your plate. Get in the habit of saving food for later. Unfortunately, starving children will not benefit from cleaning your plate.

5. **Learn to eat slowly.** It takes discipline, but failure to do so means you are likely to eat more than you need. (And we all know where those extra calories go.) Also, about twenty minutes are needed for feelings of satiation to set in. If you can avoid gobbling up food in the first few minutes, nature's satiation will make stopping easier.

6. **Avoid high-calorie drinks.** Nutritionists have long blamed sugary sodas as major contributors to America's obesity problem. But even "pure" fruit juices are no longer considered innocent. Pediatricians recognize that large servings of fruit juices contribute to overweight children. Instead, they recommend that we eat our fruits, such as apples and pears, with skins intact.

7. **Desserts—avoid when possible.** As a substitute, try small portions of fresh fruits, nuts, or cheese.

8. **Alcohol—establish a middle ground.** Not only does alcohol add significant calories to a normal meal, but the calories from alcohol are absorbed almost immediately, before those from food, making large intakes of alcohol a significant factor in weight gain.

However, since the use of alcohol is a complicated issue, with both positive and negative features, this subject will be discussed at greater length in the next chapter. For the sake of this chapter on controllable risks, I urge moderation when it comes to alcoholic drinks.

It comes as good news—which we'll see in the next chapter—that there is more that women can do in support of their own breast health.

WHAT I'D TELL MY DAUGHTER

- Exercise, exercise, exercise.
- Avoid processed foods and eat more nuts.
- It's not the fats that make you fat, it's the carbs that make you fat.
- Exercise, exercise, exercise!

✀

CHAPTER TWENTY

Alcohol, Vitamins, and Hormones: What Helps and What Hurts

O VER THE YEARS I've noticed that women who care enough about their health to appear for mammograms are grateful when I offer tips that make a long-term difference in their well-being. General good health can lower the chance of malignancies. Here are suggestions that work for most women.

ALCOHOL

I routinely ask my patients, "How many alcoholic drinks a week do you consume?" Many respond that they avoid alcohol altogether, at which I feel compelled to point out that women who consume one to two drinks a day, on average, live longer than those who don't touch it. I am not encouraging them to drink; I just want them to know the facts.

It's true—studies have shown that moderate alcohol consumption (wine, beer, and spirits) lowers the risk of death from heart disease. So if you have a family history of heart problems, you should discuss with your physician the pros and cons of moderate drinking.

That said, recent studies indicate that women who consume more than three alcoholic drinks *per week* increase their chance of developing breast cancer. In fact, women who average more than three drinks (the equivalent of a 12-ounce glass of beer, a 5-ounce glass of red wine, or 1.5 ounces of hard liquor) are at increased risk and the more that is consumed beyond that threshold, the greater the added danger.

Unfortunately, a growing body of evidence suggests that young women in particular are more vulnerable to the adverse consequences of drinking. A recent study found that even small amounts of alcohol consumed before a first pregnancy increased a woman's future chance of developing breast cancer—and the more alcohol, the greater the hazard. The studies conclude that the relatively immature breast is more vulnerable to alcohol exposure than is the case with older women.

Sadly, evidence shows that young women are drinking more and more alcohol—and, even worse, they're doing it in the most dangerous way possible: binge drinking.

BINGE DRINKING

When it comes to consuming alcohol, young women are catching up with young men. A recent study has found a 36-percent increase in female alcohol consumption between 2002 and 2012. It seems reasonable to assume that the trend among young women is still on the rise.

The biggest issue with young women is the way they drink: They usually binge on weekends. Binge drinking for women is defined as four or more drinks within a two-hour period.

Studies indicate that binge drinking involves greater hazards than drinking the same amount over a longer time period; that is, seven drinks in one night is worse than one drink a night for a week.

Unfortunately, the trend is going in the wrong direction. Hopefully, we can change this by educating young women on the perils of excessive drinking.

An added issue with alcohol, as noted in the last chapter, is that it can contribute to unwanted weight gain. Already high in calories itself, it becomes an even bigger problem when sweet mixers are added.

Further, most of us are aware that alcohol can limit inhibitions on unhealthy eating—both snacks and the meals that follow. Just think of the times you've had a couple of margaritas with friends and eagerly gobbled chips and guacamole, followed by a high-calorie Mexican meal. Nobody stops to calculate that the total calorie count probably hit 3,500.

Compounding this problem, the body metabolizes alcohol calories in preference to others. In short, this means that your body gets all the calories it needs from the liquor—while the chips go straight to your thighs.

HERE, THEN, IS A PERFECT EXAMPLE of a controllable risk factor. Whereas she can't change her family history, a woman can reduce her chances of developing breast cancer by limiting her alcohol intake.

On a more positive note, evidence suggests that taking 400 units of folic acid a day will reduce the adverse breast cancer risks associated with consuming more than three alcoholic drinks a week. It's only fitting, then, that we next discuss the issue of vitamins.

VITAMINS

In my practice, I don't push vitamins or dietary supplements. My overall advice is to eat a healthy diet, which should give you all the vitamins and minerals you need.

Recently, though, I have had a change of heart about vitamin D. An expanding body of evidence indicates that low vitamin D levels may increase a woman's chance of developing breast cancer. It also appears that women who have been diagnosed with this malignancy have a better chance of survival with adequate blood levels of vitamin D.

Since I practice in sunny southern California, I once assumed there was no need for vitamin D replacement in a region that has almost year-round sunshine. But I was wrong. I now believe that the reason for our low levels may be widespread use of sunblock (essential, of course), plus the fact that many of my patients spend most of their time indoors.

As it turns out, low vitamin D levels are a potential problem wherever you live. The solution is simple: We now encourage patients to have their vitamin D levels measured—then supplement as needed. Oral doses are readily available, inexpensive, and have a high margin of safety. I am also convinced that the threshold for normal blood levels may be too low, and that most women would be better off with higher-than-recommended levels. This is a subject that every woman should discuss with a primary care physician.

HORMONES

In chapter four, we discussed hormones related to birth control. Here the discussion revolves around a different hormonal situation: estrogen replacement for the control of menopausal symptoms.

When Premarin (which is short for "pregnant mare urine") first came on the market in the 1940s, it was considered a wonder drug. The ravages of menopause, including hot flashes, night sweats, and depression, could be eliminated with a simple pill. Another "benefit" to many women was that large doses of Premarin enhanced the size and shape of their breasts.

Unfortunately, it took thirty years to show that estrogen replacement could increase the possibility of developing uterine cancer. However, researchers soon discovered this could be prevented by adding a second hormone, progesterone, and by stopping the replacement for a few days every month to allow for a menstrual period.

More recent studies have shown that women who take combination hormone replacements after menopause for four or more years are at increased risk for developing breast cancer. Patients and their physicians were put in a bind. While hormone replacement could dramatically lower menopausal symptoms and improve bone strength, the long-term safety of such therapy came into question.

The Women's Health Initiative (WHI) recently did a significant study, involving 16,000 healthy women, on hormone replacement. The study indicated that after four years of replacement with the combination of estrogen and progesterone, called HRT (for those women who have an intact uterus), there was a small but measurable increase in the risk of breast cancer—and the risk increased with each added year of replacement hormones.

For those lucky women who go through menopause with few, if any, symptoms, the choice to avoid HRT is easy, though these women are still advised to review their options with their gynecologist.

Women who have had a previous hysterectomy are also in luck. As it turns out, recently reported studies that followed thousands of women who took estrogen replacement for thirteen years demonstrated a small reduction in breast cancer risk.

For the remaining group of women who have an intact uterus, the issue of hormone replacement is risky, as noted above. However, there may be good news on the horizon for these patients. Duavee is a new drug that provides relief of menopausal symptoms without stimulating the uterus, and it does not increase breast cancer risk. It is also beneficial in promoting bone health. We are very excited about the potential of this new drug, but it is important to remember that we lack long-term safety data.

Women who choose to stay on HRT should try to get by on the lowest possible dose that controls symptoms—while also undergoing aggressive breast cancer screening.

One of the frequent questions I get from my patients is, "Do I reduce my risk of developing breast cancer by taking bioidentical hormones [hormones that are chemically identical to those normally produced by the body]?" This question has not been adequately addressed, and an answer may be a long time coming. Until more data becomes available, it is prudent to assume that there is an equivalent risk. Like those taking synthetic hormones, women who elect to take bioidentical hormones should make an effort to get by on the lowest possible dose.

WHAT I'D TELL MY DAUGHTER

- Try to limit alcohol intake to three drinks per week.
- Avoid binge drinking.
- Know your vitamin D levels.
- Estrogen replacement alone is safe for long-term use in women who have had a hysterectomy (not safe for longer than four years for women with intact uterus), but increased breast cancer risk occurs when taking estrogen and progesterone in combination for more than four years to protect from uterine cancer.
- New drugs may make long-term combination hormone replacement safe.

"Why Me?" . . . Think DDT: The Connection Between Environmental Toxins and Cancer

ONE OF THE most challenging questions I get from newly diagnosed breast cancer patients is, "Why me?" The query typically comes from patients who have no family history of breast cancer and have, in their words, "done everything right," meaning they exercise regularly, eat properly, and maintain a healthy weight.

There is no good answer. We do know that approximately 25 percent of breast cancers occur in women who have a family history of breast or ovarian tumors. We assume that the malignancies in many of these patients are caused by gene mutations that were inherited from their parents.

Yet the enigma remains: What is the cause of cancers in the 75 percent of women who have no family history? We refer to these patients as having sporadic breast cancer. Translated, this means we simply do not know the cause.

However, a growing body of evidence suggests that exposure to chemicals in the environment, such as pesticide residue on food and by-products of plastic manufacturing, could be responsible for at least some sporadic cancers.

In 2010, the President's Cancer Panel reported that "the true burden of environmentally-induced cancers has been grossly underestimated." The report implies that our basic approach to the problem is misdirected. Currently, for a chemical to be classified as an environmental toxin, there must be "proof" that it causes harm to humans. Instead, according to the panel, a more rational approach would be to limit exposure to a toxin if there was "reasonable concern" that it could cause harm.

As expected, the chemical industry fought back, declaring that such a precautionary approach is not justified. They argued that the indiscriminate banning of chemicals could inflict an adverse impact on the economy and deny the public of the benefits associated with the introduction of new products.

With environmentalists and the industrial complex battling for control, the result has been gridlock. At present, we do not have a rational plan for dealing with existing toxins, let alone a sensible approach to new toxins being introduced into the environment each year.

To some of us, the solution is obvious: We must find a strategy to break the impasse; we need to address the issue of multiplying poisons in the environment. One approach to understanding the complexity of the problem is to review the history of what we know about environmental toxins.

The concept itself was unheard of until the late 1700s, when the English surgeon Sir Percivall Pott identified several cases of cancer of the scrotum in teenage boys who worked as chimney sweeps. Cancer of the scrotum is extremely rare, and most surgeons of that period would be unlikely to see a single case during their entire surgical careers. Finding multiple cases in boys and young men with the same occupation led Pott to conclude that there was something in the soot that was causing these malignancies.

Centuries later, scientists were able to identify the toxin responsible for scrotal cancer, what scientists now refer to as aromatic hydrocarbons.

Their presence is widespread in the environment; they are found in overcooked meats, tobacco smoke, and vehicle exhaust. Among them are known causes of lung and bladder cancers.

Pott became the first person to demonstrate that a toxin in the environment could cause cancer in humans. Since his initial observations, other "ordinary" chemicals have proven just as deadly. Two of the most widely recognized examples are asbestos, which causes the deadly cancer mesothelioma, and the aromatic hydrocarbons found in cigarette smoke, responsible for cancer of the lungs.

One of our great challenges in breast cancer care is to determine what, if any, environmental factors are responsible for the documented increase in new breast cancers over the past few decades.

One theory is that rising levels of poisonous chemicals in the environment are contributing directly to the rising rates of breast malignancies. Unfortunately, we have only limited data on humans to support this theory—though numerous scientific studies prove a direct relationship between exposure to certain toxins and the risk of developing breast cancer in laboratory animals.

Until now, there was no such study on humans. But a recently released investigation has demonstrated that exposure to the pesticide DDT in a mother could result in an increased risk of cancer in the child. It took more than fifty years to complete the study, which never would have been initiated if not for the heroic work of Rachel Carson.

RACHEL CARSON'S SONGBIRDS

Rachel Carson was a marine biologist by training and also a successful writer. In 1951, she published a best seller, *The Sea Around Us*.

In the mid-1950s she received a disturbing call from a friend describing the increasing numbers of dead songbirds that were found in fields following the spraying of DDT. A scientist at heart, Rachel was alarmed by this observation and decided to explore the issue in detail.

Because of the scientific accuracy of many of her books, Rachel was well connected with the elite scientists of the time. She grilled them about a possible adverse impact of prolonged human exposure to DDT. She found that while many scientists shared her concern, others concluded there were few, if any, risks associated with spraying. As Rachel explored the issue in greater detail, her concerns grew, as did her frustration with the lack of response from the government to protect the public from what she concluded to be a growing menace.

In desperation, she decided that the best way to get the necessary attention was to write a book exposing the dangers of prolonged exposure to DDT as well as its detrimental effects on the environment.

The title of her book was *Silent Spring*, which was a reference to the thousands of songbirds killed as a result of DDT spraying. The book was a best seller, receiving immediate attention from both the public and the government.

On multiple occasions, Rachel testified before Congress and eventually convinced members to ban the spraying of DDT. Her book became a classic. Her work on DDT gave birth to the modern green movement and led to the establishment of the EPA (Environmental Protection Agency).

It wasn't until late in her career that Rachel became suspicious that there could be a relationship between the rising rates of breast cancer and the widespread and indiscriminate spraying of DDT. Before she was able to properly address her concerns, she experienced a rapid decline in health. Ironically, she was diagnosed with metastatic breast cancer and died in 1964 at the age of fifty-six.

Despite her untimely death, Rachel's legacy lives on. In a remarkable tribute to women's health, a group of scientists inspired by her contributions decided to undertake a massive study to evaluate possible relationships between DDT and a woman's chance of developing breast cancer.

Starting in the early 1960s, thousands of pregnant women were asked to donate samples of blood to be stored for future examination.

After five decades of collecting data, the study was concluded, and in June 2015, the results were made public. A total of 118 daughters of women who participated were identified as having been diagnosed with breast cancer before the age of fifty-two.

The researchers measured the level of DDT in their mothers and compared it to levels in a much larger sample of women whose daughters did not develop malignancies. The study concluded that the daughters of mothers with the highest levels of DDT were approximately four times as likely to develop breast cancer as those with mothers at the lowest levels.

This remarkable multigenerational study represents a milestone in our understanding of environmental toxins and their influence on human breast cancer. In addition to being the first investigation to document this relationship, it also highlighted the concept of vulnerable groups. Clearly, it's the fetus that's most susceptible to DDT. In essence, it proved that levels of exposure that seem safe for an adult could be dangerous for the developing embryo.

The concept of vulnerable groups is well accepted in the field of breast care. We know, as stated in chapter two, it's perfectly safe to do yearly screening mammograms in women forty and older, but teenage girls with developing breasts are especially vulnerable to low-dose X-rays. Breast oncologists know it's relatively safe to give chemotherapy to pregnant women during the second and third trimester of a pregnancy when the fetus is fully developed. They also accept the concept of a vulnerable group—that chemo is not safe during the first trimester. In those first twelve weeks, rapidly dividing cells are forming new organs, including those that will eventually become breast tissue. What both examples demonstrate is that relatively safe levels of exposure during one period of a women's life can be highly toxic at another. Both puberty and early pregnancy serve as classic examples of vulnerable periods.

I am convinced that the DDT study will prove to be a game changer when it comes to our understanding of how environmental toxins can influence breast cancer risks. Rather than a total focus on what constitutes a safe dose, future studies must take into consideration the concept of vulnerable groups.

However, since it was banned decades ago, this issue no longer applies to DDT. But thousands of other chemicals pollute the air we breathe, the water we drink, and the food we eat.

HORMONE DISRUPTORS

The number of potential toxins is mindboggling. In attempting to get a handle on the problem, it's helpful to focus on a single group of toxins that are referred to as hormone disruptors. This group is ubiquitous in the environment, and also known to cause breast cancers in laboratory animals.

Hormone disruptors are toxins that mimic or block the action of normal hormones. By upsetting the delicate balance of hormones in the developing fetus, they produce changes that predispose the child to future breast tumors. Incidentally, DDT is classified as a hormone disruptor. Among other such disruptors lurking in the environment, the most common is bisphenol A, commonly referred to as BPA. It is found virtually everywhere—in common household plastic products like the linings of water bottles, and also in the linings of tin cans.

Laboratory studies have clearly demonstrated that exposure to BPA can cause breast cancer in animals. The FDA is adamant that the levels of exposure in our environment are safe, well below what it takes to cause breast cancer in lab animals. However, a 2012 investigation of Canadian women who work in factories that produce plastic products for cars calls into question the FDA's assumption that BPA is not an environmental threat. Women in these factories had five times the chance of developing a premenopausal breast cancer as compared to a control group. Translated, a five-times risk approaches the risk of carrying the BRCA1 gene mutation already discussed in chapter eighteen.

The FDA could well argue that this study is not applicable to the general public because levels of exposure to factory workers were so much higher than in the general environment. This may or may not be the case—but it clearly indicates that exposure to BPA can potentially increase breast cancer in humans.

One of the unanswered questions from this study is what effect elevated BPA levels will have on the daughters of factory workers. It would take decades to do a study to determine if these high levels of BPA could put fetuses at risk, as was the case with DDT. A practical approach in the meantime would be for pregnant women to limit exposure to this toxin.

We know from another study that BPA was detected in 96 percent of pregnant women who agreed to have their blood tested, but the FDA argues that the levels of BPA detected in these pregnant women were within safe limits.

Recent studies have looked more closely at the potential risk of exposing pregnant lab animals to what the FDA would consider to be within the margin of safety. These inquiries indicate that even low levels of BPA exposure during early fetal development are associated with cellular changes that predispose the developing animal fetus to an increased chance of developing a future breast cancer.

Despite the suggestive nature of this investigation, the results do not prove beyond any doubt that low levels of exposure to BPA in pregnant women lead to increased risk of breast cancer for their daughters. And it's unlikely we'll get conclusive proof in the foreseeable future.

However, the 2010 presidential report made it clear that we cannot afford to wait for conclusive evidence that any given toxin can cause breast cancer. We now have enough confirmation to express "reasonable concern." Now is the time to implement measures that will limit female exposure to known toxins.

AS IT TURNS OUT, it is remarkably easy for an individual woman to reduce her exposure to BPA—which is simply a matter of reducing contact with household plastic products. Several websites (see Bibliography) provide a step-by-step approach to making your home safe from environmental toxins. These websites provide practical advice about BPA, and outline simple steps for reducing contact with other toxins that have been proven to cause breast cancer in laboratory animals.

Here's the bigger question: What should be done to protect future generations? My review of the subject leads me to conclude that current governmental agencies are incapable of responding to this challenge.

I believe the next step is to update the 2010 presidential report. A new panel of experts should be given a mandate to outline a strategy for effectively dealing with the problem of toxins and to make specific recommendations as to what can be done to protect future generations. The newly appointed committee must have strong leadership, as well as input from our best and brightest scientists. The committee must have a clear vision of what needs to be accomplished and how they intend to get there.

We are at a turning point. We now have enough scientific data to show beyond any doubt that exposure to environmental toxins increases women's risk of developing breast cancer. Failure to act now could have major adverse consequences on future generations. Our children and our grandchildren will judge us on our response. We can ill afford to remain silent.

WHAT I'D TELL MY DAUGHTER

- Learn more about toxins in the environment and become an advocate for educating others about toxins.
- Women who are planning to become pregnant or who are in the first trimester of pregnancy should be as careful as possible about exposure to environmental toxins.

SECTION VI

After Diagnosis

CHAPTER TWENTY-TWO

Just Diagnosed: Questions You Might Have

MANY BREAST CANCER SURVIVORS, such as my co-author, have been through this scenario—cancer diagnosis, second opinions, lumpectomy, and radiation. And now, years later, they are leading lives free of cancer, as though the disease was merely a temporary interruption in their activities. This chapter covers what a woman needs to know . . . and what she can anticipate after that diagnosis.

WHAT SHOULD I EXPECT WHEN I RECEIVE "THE CALL"?

Once a breast biopsy has been performed, a woman has no alternative but to wait for the call that she fears could forever alter her life. The call could be good news, but it is almost impossible to avoid thinking about the alternative. As the hours tick by, her anxiety mounts.

Meanwhile, doctors' offices are bombarded with incoming lab reports. Often, it is difficult to determine which reports even need a callback. Yet considering the call's importance, it's remarkable how little thought doctors give to making it. This vital message for the patient is typically squeezed into a schedule that is so congested there is barely time for a lunch break, let alone extra minutes to discuss the result of a worrisome biopsy. It's not surprising that one of the more common complaints I receive from women who have just been diagnosed with cancer is the way in which they were told.

One patient's story about how she was informed she had breast cancer stands out in my memory.

THE WRONG WAY TO CONVEY BAD NEWS

Virginia was biopsied on a Monday and spent the next five days worrying about her diagnosis. By Thursday afternoon, Virginia's anxiety had reached an intolerable level. She placed several calls to the doctor's office the next day, but she still received no answer by late Friday afternoon.

That evening as she drove home from work, she knew she was about to face a long weekend of being anxious. Shortly after arriving home Friday night, however, Virginia noticed a flashing light on her kitchen phone.

With some hesitation she picked up the receiver and listened to the message. It was a one liner: "Your biopsy was positive and you need to find a breast surgeon." After a short pause, the call ended.

At least Virginia was in a safe place when she received the message. A second patient, Helen, told me she was driving on the freeway when she received a call from her doctor's office informing her that the biopsy was positive. She almost collided with oncoming traffic as she temporarily lost track of the fact that she was driving at high speed on a busy freeway.

Having heard a litany of horror stories like Virginia's and Helen's from patients treated by other doctors, I established some basic rules to inform my patients about their positive breast biopsies. (When the biopsy is negative, I simply instruct my staff to call the patient ASAP and inform her—good news, all is well.)

If the biopsy shows cancer, I always make the call myself. First, I wait until I have time to respond to the patient's immediate questions and concerns. I also make certain I've stopped to review the patient's chart in advance, so I'm familiar with the details of her case. Finally, I make it a point to give the patient a callback number to reach me if she has additional questions.

The last consideration before the call is making certain the patient is in a good place to receive it. If there is any doubt, I have the staff call first and inform her the results should be ready soon: "The doctor wants to know the best number to use and an optimum time to receive the call."

This is an issue that every woman who is scheduled to have a breast biopsy should think about. When you are making arrangements for your biopsy, make certain to provide the scheduler, or doctor's office staff, with best times and phone numbers to call.

HOW SHOULD I PREPARE FOR THE FIRST SURGICAL VISIT?

Any newly diagnosed breast cancer patient should consider in advance the questions she would like answered. One approach would be to identify her top five to ten concerns. Some women are not ready to make a list before the first visit; they want to hear from their doctor first. However, these patients still benefit from at least brainstorming a few questions and making a list—if not before that visit, then shortly afterward.

Topics discussed in this chapter can help newly diagnosed patients compile that list. There's no need to bring the entire list on your first visit. Better to review it and select the questions that seem most important at the time.

WHAT DOES MY PATHOLOGY REPORT SAY?

An important starting point is to have your doctor summarize the findings in your pathology report. Only then will you understand treatment options and prognosis. The first, and perhaps most important, thing your pathology report will tell you is what stage cancer you have. Breast cancers are divided into the following five stages:

- **Stage 0:** These cancers have not invaded the surrounding breast tissue and for the most part are considered to be curable if properly treated.
- **Stage I:** These breast cancers are small (less than 1 inch in diameter) and the cancer has not spread to the axillary (underarm) lymph nodes.
- **Stage II:** Cancers at this stage are larger than stage I, ranging from 1 inch to 2 inches in diameter. Stage II also includes women with small cancers (less than 1 inch) with limited involvement of axillary lymph nodes.
- **Stage III:** These cancers are either larger than 2 inches or have more extensive lymph node involvement.
- **Stage IV:** This stage means the cancer has spread to other organs, such as the bones or lungs. (For more details on staging, see www .breastcancer.org/symptoms/diagnosis/staging.)

Although stage is important in terms of prognosis, we know that how a tumor behaves can be even more important. For example, some large but slow-growing cancers can have an excellent prognosis, while some smaller but more aggressive malignancies can provide a poor prognosis unless treated aggressively with chemotherapy.

The pathology report will comment on the relative aggressiveness of the tumor based on the appearance of the cells under the microscope. The level of aggressiveness is broken down into three categories: low, intermediate, and high.

A second pathology report is typically received several days after the original. This follow-up describes the status of two hormone receptors, estrogen (ER) and progesterone (PR) receptors. Receptors are proteins that are normally found on the surface of cells that respond to circulating hormones in the blood stream. Cancers that are positive for the estrogen receptor (ER+) typically respond to hormone-blocking medications such as tamoxifen. PR receptors have less influence on the choice of hormone-blocking therapy, but in general the higher PR level is associated with a better prognosis.

A third receptor, called HER2+, is a growth receptor found on normal cells but seen in increased numbers (amplified) on 20 percent of all invasive breast cancers. HER2+ breast cancers tend to be fast growing, but new treatments (for example, Herceptin and Perjeta) are now available that are highly effective in dealing with these cancers.

In a third group of breast cancers the receptors are absent. These cancers are referred to as triple negative. Approximately 20 percent of breast cancers are classified this way.

WILL I HAVE CHEMO OR SURGERY FIRST?

Until recently, surgery was invariably the first step in the treatment of breast cancer. Based on the pathology report from the biopsy, the medical oncologist would then decide whether chemotherapy or hormone block was indicated before the patient had surgery. Although surgery is still the first step in most breast tumors, a growing number of women will benefit from having chemo first (also known as neoadjuvant therapy or up-front chemotherapy) and then surgery.

One of the significant advantages of giving chemo first is that it shrinks the tumor, which makes it possible to save the breast rather than doing a mastectomy.

A second advantage of "up-front" chemo is enabling the oncologist to evaluate how the cancer responds. When there is limited response, an alternative combination of drugs can be used.

Third, there is always the possibility that the up-front chemo will eliminate cancer cells in the axillary (armpit) lymph nodes, meaning less lymph node surgery. By reducing the number of excised lymph nodes, we also reduce the chance of a swollen arm that can occur months to years after such surgery. Arm swelling after lymph node surgery is referred to as lymphedema.

Triple negative and HER2+ patients typically benefit from receiving chemo first, as do the more advanced estrogen-receptor-positive breast cancers. At our center, the fallback rule about giving chemo up-front is quite simple. If our oncologist concludes that a patient will benefit from chemo, we prefer to give it before going to surgery.

WILL I NEED A SENTINEL NODE BIOPSY?

Prior to the mid-1990s, patients with invasive breast cancers routinely underwent the removal of all the armpit (axillary) lymph nodes, which frequently led to unpleasant symptoms such as pain, restriction of motion, and the feared complication of lymphedema. Yet in most patients with early cancer, the lymph nodes were not involved. The only benefit to these patients was the knowledge that their cancer was confined to their breast.

It is now standard policy to remove the first few draining lymph nodes. We know that if these nodes are negative it is unnecessary to remove the rest, because those further along the chain will also be negative. Consequently, we refer to these nodes as the sentinel lymph nodes, since marauding cancer visits them first.

It is quite easy to identify the sentinel nodes. The most common way is to inject the breast with a radioactive material (Technetium-99m) prior to surgery. This substance travels through the lymph channels and ends up in the sentinel lymph nodes. The nodes can be readily detected with a Geiger counter–like device that shows increasing numbers on a screen as the probe nears its target. These identified nodes will then be removed by the surgeon.

Since the sentinel node biopsy procedure has become the standard approach to determining the status of the lymph nodes in patients with early breast cancer, the incidence of lymphedema or arm swelling has dropped precipitously. Another major advance is the availability of a new technology that can detect early lymphedema before the swelling is noticeable. The new product, known as L-Dex, is accurate in detecting early lymphedema when it is still reversible. The L-Dex machine is now used routinely in all of our patients who have undergone lymph node removal.

WILL I NEED RADIATION?

Radiation therapy is used to kill any lingering cancer cells that might remain after a lumpectomy. In cases of more advanced cancers, radiation sometimes follows a mastectomy (both lumpectomies and mastectomies will be discussed in chapter twenty-four). Radiation therapy is performed by a radiation oncologist.

In the past, radiation following a lumpectomy meant exposing the entire breast to radiation. The treatments, given daily except for weekends, usually lasted six to seven weeks. Whole breast radiation, as it is usually called, is still the standard therapy for most invasive breast cancers. However, shorter courses of radiation are now being used for smaller and less aggressive breast cancers.

In selected cases, radiation can be given at the time of surgery. The procedure is referred to as IORT (intra-operative radiation therapy). With other patients, a short course of radiation can be given following surgery. This procedure is referred to as PBI or partial breast irradiation. The procedure is typically done a few weeks following surgery and requires five days of twice-daily radiation.

It has recently been established in a study that women over seventy with small low-grade cancers can safely avoid radiation (because of the lack of benefit in term recurrence or survival rates), but they still need to take hormone-blocking pills.

WHAT DO I NEED TO KNOW
ABOUT MARGINS?

Understanding the concept of margins is essential to grasping why some women are good candidates for saving their breast and others are not. The basic idea is fairly simple: When performing a lumpectomy for breast cancer, it is essential to remove not just the entire malignancy but also a rim of normal tissue—called a margin—surrounding the tumor. Failure to do so results in increased rates of local recurrence.

In the past, what constitutes a safe margin was an issue of major controversy. There is now a growing consensus that the margin is clear as long as there is no invasive cancer at the edge of the lumpectomy specimen. If the pathologist does see tumor cells on the edge of the specimen, a second surgery is required. The issue of what is an adequate margin width in cases of non-invasive cancer is still being debated, but we prefer to obtain a 2mm margin in most cases.

SHOULD I SEE A PLASTIC SURGEON?

A plastic surgeon should be an integral part of any multidisciplinary treatment team. It's important for women who might benefit from reconstruction to be seen as soon as possible to help coordinate care with the breast surgeon. The details of what the plastic surgeon can add to the overall treatment plan will be discussed in chapter twenty-four.

WILL MY CASE BE PRESENTED TO A MULTIDISCIPLINARY CONFERENCE?

The multidisciplinary team (also referred to as a tumor board) typically includes physicians from several disciplines, including radiology, pathology, breast surgery, plastic surgery, medical oncology, and radiation oncology. Other members of the team may include members from a research department, as well as nutritionists and psychosocial support personnel.

Most conferences take place on a weekly basis, and usually the patient is not present. Ideally, all newly diagnosed breast cancers should be presented to the conference. Even after many years of reviewing cases in our multidisciplinary group, I am impressed at how often the patient benefits from the members' collective input.

When a multidisciplinary conference is not available, the patient should ask the surgeon how his or her colleagues address the issue of coordinating care.

BEFORE SURGERY, DO I NEED A BREAST MRI?

The value of the MRI in assisting treatment decisions is one of the more controversial issues in breast care. Some well-known surgical experts suggest that MRIs are rarely indicated because they can lead to unnecessary biopsies and treatment delays. In addition, some studies suggest that women who have MRIs are more likely to end up with a mastectomy.

We believe the MRI is very useful in treatment planning, and we use it on most women with dense breasts or when the extent of the cancer is not clearly demonstrated on the mammogram or ultrasound. When tumors are easily identified in women with primarily fatty breasts, we usually forgo an MRI.

DO I NEED GENETIC TESTING?

As discussed in chapter eighteen, our current policy is to offer genetic testing to all of our newly diagnosed breast cancer patients.

SHOULD I PARTICIPATE IN A RESEARCH TRIAL, IF OFFERED?

There are two reasons why every woman should participate in clinical trials when available. The first is quite simple: You may gain access to a drug that will save your life (see chapter twenty-eight).

The second is the benefit of giving back to the community. If it were not for clinical trials, we would still be doing radical mastectomies, and lifesaving targeted therapies such as Herceptin would not be available.

Most of the major advances in breast cancer care came about because of patient participation in these trials.

The tagline from our nonprofit research foundation (Cancer Research Collaboration, or CRC) is worth remembering: "Without research there will be no cure."

SHOULD I PURSUE ALTERNATIVE MEDICINE?

I am not an advocate of alternative medicine, which substitutes alternative treatments for standard medical care (i.e., surgery, chemo, and radiation). I am a strong advocate for complementary medicine (i.e., tai chi, yoga, and massage therapy) added to standard medical care. In my experience it is often very effective in lowering stress levels.

THE DOWNSIDE OF ALTERNATIVE MEDICINE

Morgan (not her real name) was forty-two years old when she found a lump the size of a small egg in her left breast. Her first mammogram showed a large cancer with at least one suspicious lymph node under her arm. A core needle biopsy was positive for both the breast lump and the lymph node.

She was a biologist by training and had two young daughters. She wanted to get started on therapy ASAP. On her second visit she appeared with an obvious change in attitude. She told me God came to her in a dream—telling her if she had faith in Him, her cancer would go away.

I was stunned. She had an aggressive cancer that needed immediate medical attention, but she'd recently discussed her dilemma with a "cancer naturalist" who supported her decision to pray as long as she was willing to follow nutritional recommendations.

To my surprise, she still wanted me to follow her at regular intervals. In retrospect, I concluded this was to prove to me that the combination of faith in God and a proper diet could make the cancer go away.

I told her I would continue to see her if she would sign a letter stating she was fully aware of the consequences of not following standard medical advice. To be sure she fully understood her decision, I included a line in the letter that indicated she was aware that by not continuing with standard treatment guidelines, her two young daughters could grow up without a mother.

She was buried two years later.

I share Morgan's story with my patients who are considering alternative therapy, but, unfortunately, it usually doesn't help.

On the other hand, I strongly embrace the concept of complementary therapy. We've had patients on the verge of stopping chemo because of severe nausea and other side effects. Alternatively, we've had others with persistent post-operative incisional pains that were resistant to standard treatment. Herbal medicine and acupuncture have sometimes worked miracles in counteracting the side effects from chemotherapy and surgery.

WHAT ABOUT SUPPORT SERVICES?

Most breast care centers have support programs, and it's advisable for newly diagnosed patients to participate in them (see chapter twenty-eight).

One of the most valuable forms of support is group sessions with other newly diagnosed breast cancer patients. The most effective groups are usually led by someone with special training in support techniques. Just being around other women who are undergoing a similar journey makes it easier for patients to deal with the complexity of their care.

For patients where support services are not readily available, help can be found on the web (see Appendix II).

DO I NEED A SECOND OPINION?

This could be the most important question you can ask. As it turns out, many women in the United States will not get the same treatment that I would advise for a family member. If you have even the slightest doubt about your care, get a second opinion. The reasons for doing so are explained in the next chapter.

CHAPTER TWENTY-THREE

Who Needs a Second Opinion—and Why?

Newly diagnosed breast cancer patients are often asked by family and friends, "Are you getting a second opinion?" It's a question with merit. Recent studies have demonstrated a worrisome number of errors in pathology reports from breast biopsies.

Some women, for example, are told they have breast cancer when in fact their biopsy is benign. Others get the exciting news that they don't have a malignancy, only to learn later that the report was wrong and they do have cancer.

An erroneous pathology report is a problem of major proportions. Our treatment decisions are directly based on that information. If the diagnosis is wrong, our treatment recommendations will also be wrong.

Diagnostic errors in breast biopsy specimens are of such concern that in 2006 the Susan G. Komen Breast Cancer Foundation published a comprehensive white paper detailing the magnitude of the problem and providing extensive recommendations for improving accuracy.

Yet a decade later, the worrisome issue still existed. An article in the June 2015 issue of *The Journal of the American Medical Association* concluded that there are still significant problems with accuracy in breast biopsy pathology reports. The study concluded that pathologists did a fairly good job of diagnosing invasive breast cancer, where an accurate diagnosis was made in 97 percent of the cases. However, the investigation reported a 25 percent error rate for interpreting slides that contained ductal carcinoma in situ (DCIS) or other high-risk changes that were associated with an increased risk of developing cancer in the future.

Such a large rate of errors seems almost inconceivable. How could it be that one in four women who receive a diagnosis of a high-risk biopsy could be given inaccurate information? Even more disturbing is the 3 percent error rate for invasive breast cancers. The conclusion is obvious: There is an urgent need to improve the quality of pathology reports. However, achieving this goal is challenging.

HOW DOES PATHOLOGY WORK?

In an attempt to illustrate just how difficult it is for a pathologist to make an accurate diagnosis, I will briefly describe the basic steps.

I am not a pathologist, but I did do a three-month rotation in pathology during my surgical residency. I learned firsthand just how demanding the job of the pathologist can be when evaluating breast biopsy specimens. In those days, the pathologist received a specimen from the surgeon who had just removed a breast lump from a woman who was still under general anesthesia. The pathologist was responsible for making a rapid decision as to whether the lump was malignant or benign. If the lump was judged malignant, the next step was a mastectomy. If the lump was labeled benign, the surgeon would simply close the incision.

The pathologist would freeze tissue received from the surgeon so that it could be quickly processed. It was then placed on a slide for review. In the vast majority of cases, the pathologist made an accurate diagnosis. Occasionally, though, he or she could not make a definitive diagnosis, in which case the surgeon was informed and told to wait a few days for a final diagnosis. In the next few days the tissue would undergo a series of processing steps, intended to create permanent sections that show greater cellular detail and are easier to interpret than those that are frozen.

Today, frozen sections are rarely used to make a diagnosis of cancer. Now the abnormal breast tissue is sampled with a core needle, then placed in a formalin solution and sent to pathology for processing and, ultimately, for permanent sections. Unlike in that earlier era, the pathologist is no longer under extreme time pressure to make a diagnosis. The final report is usually available in two to three days.

In most cases, it is relatively easy to make an accurate diagnosis on permanent sections. However, there are some cases in which the distinction between benign and premalignant or between premalignant and malignant can be quite subtle. It is here, in these borderline cases, where many of the diagnostic errors are made.

In an attempt to better describe what is meant by borderline lesions, it's best to start with a simple description of a normal cell. Normal breast cells are round or rectangular and have a small, round black spot in each center called the nucleus. Cancer cells, however, are usually irregular in shape and the central nucleus is enlarged. The cancer cells often grow into abnormal groups or clumps, rather than forming the microscopic patterns of normal breast tissue.

The first observable step in the cell's transitioning from normal to cancerous is the evidence of greater cellular growth within the breast ducts. To the pathologist the cells look normal, but there's a relative increase in numbers. This condition is referred to as hyperplasia and is not associated with an increased risk of developing future cancer. As the transition to malignancy progresses, the cells continue to increase in number and become more crowded. The nucleus often becomes larger and more irregular. These cellular changes are referred to as atypia. Women who have atypical breast biopsies *are* at increased risk of future cancer. As changes progress, a threshold is finally reached in which the cells can be appropriately classified as malignant.

In the early stages, these cancer cells are confined to the inside of the breast ducts (the DCIS mentioned earlier). DCIS is a cancer, but it is a potentially curable form. The final step occurs when the cells break through the lining of the duct and invade the surrounding breast tissue. In the earliest phases of invasion, only a few cells break through, a condition referred to as micro-invasion. It can be so subtle that it can be easily overlooked by the pathologist.

These basic principles sound simple enough, but, in actual practice, diagnosis is far tougher than I have outlined. Pathologists usually agree on the diagnosis when cellular patterns fit neatly into one category or the other . . . but in difficult cases the cells may be at a transition point from benign to premalignant or from premalignant to malignant, which is where we see significant disagreement among pathologists. For example, what one pathologist might call severe hyperplasia another may call mild atypia. If, in the same example, the pathologist made the diagnosis of atypia, the woman would be informed that she was at increased risk of developing breast cancer and would be encouraged to begin hormone-blocking therapy.

IN THE 1950S, Dr. David Page, one of the world's leading authorities on the subject of breast pathology, spearheaded a thirty-year study attempting to settle the debate by establishing a set of criteria on how to classify high-risk lesions. Dr. Page began collecting cases of women who had a previous high-risk breast biopsy but refused to have surgery to remove the area of concern. He followed thousands of women for several decades. Among them he identified a large number of women who went on to develop breast cancer.

With that evidence at hand, he studied the original biopsies of those now cancer-diagnosed women. Eventually, he was able to establish criteria for differentiating an abnormal-appearing cellular pattern that doesn't put a woman at increased risk from a similar-looking cellular pattern that does—one that I learned about when one of my patients became proactive about her own diagnosis.

A PATIENT LEADS THE WAY TO BETTER DIAGNOSES

Carole Follman was a friend, a community leader, and a strong supporter of many local charities. I had known Carole and her family for years. She considered me a trusted physician.

She was also a long-term patient. I would see her yearly on the same day she got her mammogram. A few years ago her mammogram showed a new cluster of calcifications. The results of a core needle biopsy were interpreted as atypia (atypical ductal hyperplasia, or ADH) and an open biopsy confirmed the diagnosis of "extensive atypia." Initially relieved when the biopsy showed no evidence of cancer, she was not at all pleased with my recommendations.

As is standard for women who are diagnosed with atypia, I urged that she stop her estrogen and go on tamoxifen to lower her future risk of developing cancer. Carole was not a happy camper. She made it abundantly clear that she did not want to go on tamoxifen because of concerns about side effects.

She was also well connected to many leaders in our medical community. One of her closest friends was a general surgeon who'd been Richard Nixon's personal physician when he was president. Her doctor friend knew of a world-class pathologist who specialized in breast cancer, and suggested she take her slides to him for a second opinion.

The pathologist was Dr. Lowell Rogers, who trained at Vanderbilt University under the direction of Dr. David Page . . . the same Dr. Page who had established criteria for differentiating abnormal-appearing cellular patterns that are not suggestive of increased breast cancer risk from similar-looking patterns that are associated with an increased risk. Dr. Rogers reviewed Carole's slides and came to the conclusion that she did not have atypical changes on her biopsy. He did see what he called advanced hyperplastic changes, but he was convinced the cellular changes were not sufficient to meet his criteria for atypia. Using the criteria established by Dr. Page's study, Dr. Rogers was able to say with certainty that Carole was not at increased risk and did not need to go on tamoxifen. Twenty years later, she remains cancer free.

Dr. Page's criteria would have made classifying high-risk lesions much easier if the pathology community had immediately recognized the study's conclusions. But, as is so often the case, egos got in the way. Other well-recognized pathologists had their own ideas about how to classify various high-risk lesions. As a result, an ongoing debate erupted about who was right and who was wrong. At that time, it was possible for the same set of slides to be sent to three senior pathologists, resulting in three different opinions on the diagnosis.

Before Carole's biopsy, I assumed our hospital had a world-class department of pathology. After all, they had all been trained at some of America's most prestigious centers. When Carole brought Dr. Rogers's results back to me, it became immediately clear that we needed to make major changes in our department of pathology. We needed to adopt the criteria set forth by Dr. Page to classify our high-risk breast biopsy specimens.

I discussed this with our chief of pathology. At first, he was reluctant to make any commitments. I explained to him that Carole insisted on action, indicating that she was prepared to go public if the issue was not resolved. Our department head finally agreed that changes must be made but was unsure how to go about it—especially with a group that had been doing things the same way for decades.

I discussed the dilemma with Carole. She said it was simple: Just bring Dr. Page to Orange County. This seemed a suggestion that would go nowhere—Dr. Page was incredibly busy and could not possibly have the time to properly address our needs—but, to my surprise, Dr. Page was not only willing to come and help but he suggested we put on a symposium for the pathologists in Orange and surrounding counties.

The symposium proved to be a real eye-opener. Each participating pathologist was asked to bring slides from one or more challenging cases for the group to review. The slides were projected on a screen, and each doctor was given a device to check off his interpretation of the slides from a list of options. The choices from each physician were tabulated in a central computer and the results displayed in a graphic format on television monitors.

The pattern was similar for the thirty or more slides that were reviewed. The spectrum of choices ran the gamut from hyperplasia to atypia to DCIS. In some cases, the majority of the participants agreed with the selection made by Dr. Page, but in most cases they didn't.

The conclusions were obvious to every participant. An incredible inconsistency appeared among practicing pathologists when it came to interpreting difficult breast biopsy slides. After the conference was over, we were all overwhelmed, but we were also inspired by the program's success.

Dr. Page stayed with us for a week, during which time we appointed one of our senior pathologists to take on the role of director of breast pathology. He was required to spend several weeks at Vanderbilt working with Dr. Page. He also agreed to implement a new policy at our hospital in which he would do a second read on all breast biopsy slides.

At the end of the week we met at Carole's house to thank Dr. Page and celebrate the huge progress that had been made in such a short time. Rather than taking credit for the project, Dr. Page gave all the credit to Carole. He informed us that in his entire career he had never heard of a patient taking such an aggressive role in coercing a hospital to upgrade the quality of its pathology department. Come to think of it, no one else in the room was aware of a similar situation. We all agreed that Carole was the real hero.

The lesson learned from this experience is that a patient cannot take for granted that her biopsy report is accurate. In cases in which the diagnosis is obviously benign or obviously malignant, a second opinion is usually not needed. However, if there is any question, it is easy to get a second opinion. The cost of the slide review is in the range of $200 to $300, and insurance will often cover part or all of it.

My recommendations for the top three choices for obtaining a second opinion on your path report:

1. Vanderbilt: Vanderbilt-Ingram Cancer Center—www.vanderbilt health.com/cancer/36570
2. Breastlink—www.breastlink.com/services/breast-cancer-second -opinion
3. Michael D. Lagios—www.breastcancerconsultdr.com/second_ opinion/second_opinion.html

NOT ONLY THE PATH REPORT CAN BE WRONG

It would be wonderful if all we had to do to ensure optimal breast care was to send biopsy slides for a second opinion. As it turns out, mistakes are common in virtually every aspect of breast cancer care. Several recent studies have documented that the same kinds of errors in judgment occurring within the pathology department also take place in all the other departments that deal with the newly diagnosed patient.

Recent studies have examined what happens to women who get a second opinion. They conclude that treatment recommendations from the center providing the second opinion differ from the original recommendation in up to half of all cases. In some instances, the differences of opinion were small, but in a disturbingly large percentage major alterations of the original treatment plan were recommended.

In our second opinion program we see instances in which the original mammogram missed a second cancer. We also commonly find women for whom a mastectomy was recommended, when she was actually a good candidate for breast conservation. One of the most common mistakes we encounter is physicians telling patients they need immediate surgery when, in fact, what they really need is chemo first to shrink the tumor and take care of any cells that have broken off from the original site and entered the patient's bloodstream (see chapter twenty-two).

THE PATIENT WHO is seriously considering a second opinion should be aware of a few issues. The first is timing. It takes time to gather your pathology slides and copies of your imaging to take with you when you meet with the second opinion team. The sooner you make the decision, the better. For most, the extra few days are of no concern. Yet there are some cases of aggressive breast cancers that are in urgent need of chemotherapy. When these women call us for a second opinion we direct them to our oncology department and attempt to start chemo as soon as possible.

Also, a patient should be prepared for conflicting recommendations between the first and second opinions. Do you get a third opinion or stay with the group that gives you the most confidence and peace of mind? This is a judgment call that only the patient can make. But it is important to remember that the clock is ticking and decisions must be made without excessive delay.

A final issue of concern is for women in rural areas where the closest comprehensive center is hours away. One option is to have slides and images sent to a center that is willing to render a second opinion without the patient being present. In some centers video conferencing is also available. Patients can now get extra advice without leaving home.

Despite the negative examples presented in this chapter, there is reason for optimism. The College of American Pathologists is committed to improving the accuracy of the path report by providing additional training to practicing pathologists. The American Society of Breast Surgeons has done an incredible job of providing advanced training to breast care surgeons.

Other medical societies, including the American College of Radiology and the American Society of Clinical Oncology, are leaders in the field of improving the quality of breast care. The two have made notable progress in providing advanced education to radiologists and oncologists.

Finally, women themselves offer a reason for optimism. More and more I see engaged patients who are aware of the need for a proactive approach when dealing with their personal breast care.

WHILE SO FAR this chapter thoroughly covers the topic of second opinions after a cancer diagnosis, what do you do when you suspect something might be amiss in one of your breasts, but a mammogram says you're okay and even your primary care doctor can't find anything wrong?

From my co-author, Maralys Wills, I've learned what it means for a woman to be skeptical of good news that seems out of line with her instincts—with a sense that "something is not quite right." Her story is about stubbornly taking charge of your own health, even in the face of professional opinions that, at the time, seem good enough so that anyone could be lured into false complacency. Maralys trusted her instincts and got a second opinion that may have been lifesaving.

A WOMAN'S STUBBORNNESS PAYS OFF

Maralys was not one of the younger women whose cancer surprised them. Instead, she was in her early seventies . . . active, playing tennis, and, except for arthritis, in pretty good health. For years she'd been something of a health nut, making sure most of her food was nutritious ("except for the occasional See's candy") and making time for almost-daily exercise, on the treadmill or otherwise.

It was during recovery from knee replacement that she had the sensation that "something wasn't right" in her left breast. She says, "It was all so subtle. My husband brought my bra to wear in the hospital bed, and that night I forgot to take it off. Next morning my left breast felt 'different.' Different is what alerted me to take action."

Though not yet walking well, she asked her husband to take her for a mammogram the second week she was home from the hospital—her first trip out of the house. The news from the screening was good. To the radiologist, everything looked normal. And here's where her "German stubbornness," as she calls it, came into play. For most women, most of the time, "good" and "normal" are all they need to hear in a report. Meaning no more mammograms for another year.

But because of her "something's not right" feeling, doubts remained. She says, "I guess I'm one of those people who have to be convinced ten times over."

She scheduled a visit with her internist, who did a physical exam and found nothing. But he did say, "If you still have doubts, you should probably go see an expert—Dr. John West." So she did.

Before I could make a decision, she said, "Shouldn't we remove it, whatever it is?" and I agreed. However, I expected the lump to be benign.

I especially didn't expect cancer. But that's what it was. I removed the lump surgically, and I admitted that the cancer had surprised me as much as it did her.

Later she said, "I'd already recited to myself all the reasons it was probably nothing. There was no cancer in my family. I'd had six children and nursed them all. I'd taken pretty good care of my health. From all my past reading, I didn't fit the pattern."

I said, "There is no pattern. Your biggest risk factor is simply being a woman."

Yet she was lucky after all. The pathology report called the tumor slow growing and non-aggressive.

With sentinel lymph node removal, pathology showed the cancer hadn't spread. She began a course of radiation and reported back to me, "I had zero side effects. I was never tired, never in pain. The only nuisance was simply appearing a number of weeks for radiation."

Now, ten years later, a scar-tissue lump lingers in that breast, but her mammograms, and even an MRI, show no evidence of cancer.

Maralys's story serves as a powerful reminder. When the question "Who needs a second opinion?" is considered, the answer is simple: *Any woman who thinks she does.*

WHAT I'D TELL MY DAUGHTER

- Every woman who has been diagnosed with breast cancer should consider getting a second opinion.
- Pathology second opinions should be considered when the biopsy shows atypia or DCIS.
- If you think you need a second opinion, get one!

※

CHAPTER TWENTY-FOUR

Mastectomy Versus Lumpectomy

MASTECTOMY THEN AND NOW

When I started my surgical practice in the early 1970s, radical mastectomy was the standard treatment for women with breast cancer, which meant at the time—and still does—that the entire breast (including the chest wall muscles and all of the axillary lymph nodes) was removed. This surgery will be described in greater detail in chapter twenty-five.

In that era of the 1970s, mammography was not widely available—in fact, it was just getting off the ground. Women would come to us when they or their doctors found a breast lump, which was usually the size of a walnut or larger. By the time we saw them in the office, the diagnosis was fairly obvious. Cancer lumps were hard, irregular, and often attached to the skin. Non-cancerous lumps (benign mounds) were usually smooth, round, and mobile.

Despite the fact that it was fairly easy to tell which nodules were cancerous, all patients with lumps were told that surgical removal under general anesthesia was required to make an accurate diagnosis. The pathologist would do a frozen section while they were asleep. If the biopsy revealed cancer, we did a mastectomy.

We told our patients if they woke up with a small Band-Aid–like dressing they could be assured the biopsy was not cancer. Patients with cancer awoke with large bulky dressings and cumbersome wound drains. No wonder there was such intense fear of going to the doctor with a breast lump.

Much has been accomplished in the past few decades to make life easier for women with a breast mass. One major positive step is our ability to make an accurate diagnosis without taking women to surgery.

We now take a small sample from the suspicious area with a needle, which provides all the information we need for an accurate diagnosis. The needle biopsy is done under local anesthesia, and takes fewer than thirty minutes to perform in an outpatient setting.

If it proves to be benign, it can either be followed clinically or removed through a small cosmetic incision. If the biopsy shows cancer, the patient is presented to a tumor board, where a panel of experts discuss the findings and make treatment recommendations.

Although making the diagnosis with a core needle biopsy is considered the standard of care, there are still many areas in the United States where women are not given this option. Instead, they are taken directly to surgery to have the entire mass removed. This is simply bad medicine. It complicates the future treatment of patients who are diagnosed with breast cancer and subjects women with benign masses to unnecessary surgery.

Though core needle biopsies were a major advancement in breast care, an even greater step forward was the elimination of radical mastectomy as the primary treatment of choice for women with breast cancer.

The history of how surgeons learned to treat such women dates back thousands of years. An ancient Egyptian papyrus was the first known document to comment on the treatment of breast cancer. The advice was simple: "If you find a cold hard breast mass," which was their description of an advanced cancer, "leave it alone." The papyrus went on to describe how draining an abscess could be lifesaving in women with a breast infection.

The advice from the papyrus about avoiding breast surgery was reaffirmed in a subsequent dictum from the ancient Greeks. Two hundred years before the birth of Christ, Greek physicians first introduced the concept of *primum non nocere*, which, translated, means, "First, do no harm." For the next 2,000 years of recorded history, surgeons failed to follow this dictum in their efforts to treat patients' breast cancers. During that period, surgical care typically did cause more harm than good.

It was Dr. William Halsted who, in 1882, developed the first operation that actually benefited women. What Halsted accomplished was not so much a curative operation but a procedure that dramatically reduced the chances of a cancer recurring in the same area. The issue of "local recurrence" following surgery was a common and dreaded complication in the era before the "Halsted Radical Mastectomy."

The radical mastectomy was the first operation ever developed by an American surgeon; as a result, the procedure bears his name, and Dr. Halsted was awarded the title of "Father of American Surgery" for this and many other accomplishments.

SAVING A BREAST: LUMPECTOMY

By the time I started my training, Dr. Halsted was held in god-like reverence. No surgical resident would dare consider taking issue with Halsted's advice. But despite his incredible personal reputation, a few surgeons were questioning the value of the radical mastectomy.

One of these renegades was a young Italian surgeon named Umberto Veronesi. Somehow, in the 1960s, Dr. Veronesi was able to convince his peers in Europe to participate in a study comparing the long-term results of mastectomy to the results of just removing the lump and irradiating the breast, a procedure we now refer to as breast-conserving surgery (BCS) or lumpectomy.

Following Veronesi's lead, a similar study was done in the United States under the supervision of Dr. Bernard Fisher. Both studies drew the same conclusion: Survival was identical for women undergoing mastectomy as compared to women who had only a lumpectomy plus radiation.

I started my practice in 1973. At that time community surgeons were not giving women the option of saving their breasts. It was time for a change in attitudes, but, as it turned out, old habits were hard to break.

Our local surgeons were making significant progress in caring for women with breast lumps and had already abandoned the one-step approach to diagnosing and treating breast cancer. No longer were women with nodules required to sign a consent form for mastectomy and undergo a general anesthetic to get a diagnosis. By this time, surgeons were removing the lump as a first step. If it was found to be malignant, a mastectomy was next.

This two-step approach relieved some of the anxiety about going to the doctor for a new breast lump. It also allowed women who tested positive to get a second opinion. It was just such a request for a second opinion that prompted me to do my first lumpectomy. Although I was convinced that lumpectomy was a safe alternative to mastectomy, I did not want to be the first surgeon in the community to do it. I had already rubbed the medical community the wrong way by criticizing how emergency care was being handled. It was too early in my surgical career to have a second strike against me. It took a strong-willed woman, Barbara, to finally convince me to do the right thing.

A VERY DETERMINED PATIENT

One morning when I was seeing patients in my office, my staff received a call from a very anxious patient. Carly had been diagnosed with breast cancer and wanted to be seen immediately. The receptionist explained that the office was already overbooked, but we would try to squeeze her in the next day if possible.

In desperation, she informed the staff that if she could not get an appointment that day, she would camp outside my door and stay there until I saw her. I gave in. After all, who really needs a lunch break?

A quick review of her case indicated she would be an ideal candidate for saving her breast. Her cancer was small and located in an area that made it easy to remove without causing major change to the shape of her breast.

It was just the kind of case I was looking for. When I told her I would do her surgery within the week, she showed immediate relief and gave me a big hug.

Carly's surgery and radiation went without a hitch, and she had a wonderful result. Thirty years later she is still alive, happy, and cancer-free. I look back on her case with pride, knowing I was, to my knowledge, the first surgeon in the area to cure a breast cancer without a mastectomy.

Not all cases were as straightforward as Carly's. As is usually the situation, we went through a learning curve. It was not always easy to get clearance around the tumor. We often had to do a second or third operation to ensure removal of the microscopic extensions of the malignancy. The cosmetic results were usually less favorable when a return to the operating room was required.

Over time, surgery became more effective in terms of clearing margins on the first attempt. As surgeons improved their techniques, so did the radiation oncologists who developed methods leading to fewer skin changes, less hardening of the breast, and less damaging radiation scatter to other organs, such as the heart or lungs.

Although I will never forget my first experience with Carly, Kim's case also stands out as an example of just how good it gets when we use modern approaches to save the breast.

LUMPECTOMY—AS GOOD AS IT GETS

Kim was in her early forties when she was diagnosed with an early-stage breast cancer. She was a good candidate for BCS. On the first attempt, we were able to remove the cancer with clear margins. Subsequently, she underwent six weeks of radiation.

I saw her in the office about a decade after her original breast cancer surgery. It was one of those typical busy office days. She'd had a mammogram an hour before her appointment, and it was completely normal. I was in a bit of a rush. I briefly scanned the mammogram report, and then went directly to the physical exam without reviewing her previous records.

When I first examined her breasts, they both looked perfectly normal. She'd had a previous benign biopsy on one side and breast-conserving surgery on the other and at this visit she presented with two well-healed incisions.

The "problem" was, I could not tell by looking at her which breast had been operated on for cancer. Rather than return to the chart for the answer, I simply asked her, "Which side was your breast cancer on?" If ever I needed a reminder of just how good BCS could be, this was the case.

WHY SO MANY MASTECTOMIES?

In my mind, the controversy of mastectomy versus lumpectomy was over, and breast conservation won.

Or did it? Despite the obvious benefits of breast conservation, there appears to be a growing trend for women who are candidates for breast conservation to elect to have a mastectomy. Even more surprising is the observation that, at the time of their mastectomy, some of these women are also choosing to have prophylactic mastectomies, which means removal of the opposite, normal—meaning cancer-free—breast.

Breast conservation is considered the standard of care for most women when it is technically possible to do so; lumpectomies are relatively easy, outpatient surgical procedures. Recovery is quick and complications are uncommon. Furthermore, the cosmetic results are usually excellent. Thus mastectomy has become the fallback procedure . . . or has it?

Just when you think you know all there is to know about surgery, things change, sometimes so slowly that you are not even aware a shift is taking place.

I remember a time, in the not too distant past, when I was going through a rather mechanical explanation of surgical options to a patient who was diagnosed with a small cancer. She was an ideal candidate for BCS, and I just assumed she would immediately recognize the benefits of saving her breast.

It came as a shock to me when I finished my presentation and she said, "I want a mastectomy." I initially felt it was my responsibility to make a better breast-saving case, but my instincts told me she had already made up her mind. She seemed relieved when I told her I was willing to do it her way.

I felt embarrassed as I presented her case to our weekly tumor board. After reviewing all the details, the group came to the obvious conclusion that lumpectomy was the procedure of choice. When I told our experts the patient was adamant about mastectomy, they seemed puzzled. I got the distinct feeling some colleagues were suspicious that I hadn't given the patient an adequate explanation of the benefits of BCS.

In the next several months I observed other women who were ideal candidates for lumpectomy yet chose mastectomy. At first, I thought this was just a coincidence. I also considered the alternative explanation—that I was overreacting. A few outliers were having a significant impact on my memory. This was not a trend; it was more of an unusual cluster of patients who were going against standard medical advice, or at least that was my current conclusion.

My second clue that attitudes toward mastectomy were changing became apparent when I was discussing surgical options with a physician colleague recently diagnosed with a small breast cancer. After a lengthy discussion of her various treatment options, she looked at me with steely eyes and said, "I want 'em both off."

I found her blunt response unsettling. She simply cut me off when I suggested she at least consider other options; she made it clear no further discussion was needed. This physician's strong bias toward mastectomy prompted me to ponder how women perceive the two alternatives of surgical care. To many, if not most, there is a distinct advantage to saving their breasts. They are willing to do whatever it takes to keep them, as long as it is safe.

Others have a much different attitude about surgical options. As one patient said, "The breasts are for attracting men and feeding babies." I knew she was exaggerating, but her point was that some women consider the breasts to be a liability when they have been diagnosed with cancer. For them, mastectomy is the option that gives them the greatest peace of mind.

The fact that a female physician, who was an excellent candidate for lumpectomy, elected mastectomy instead prompted me to review my experience with treating other physicians who had a similar diagnosis. In doing so, I was able to identify a dozen physicians on whom I'd operated in the past few decades. Of the twelve, all but one chose mastectomy. The single exception was a radiation oncologist.

ALTHOUGH I FINALLY became convinced that there was evidence that more women who were candidates for lumpectomy were now opting for mastectomy, I was careful to keep my mouth shut—very unusual for me. I was well aware that any statement that failed to recognize the superiority of BCS would be considered heresy by my colleagues.

One more event further supported that I was right about changing attitudes in some women toward the relative benefits of mastectomy over breast conservation. The event was a regional meeting of physicians who specialized in all aspects of breast cancer care. Approximately seventy participants attended the conference, more than half of whom were women.

One of the topics was the issue of surgeons performing too many mastectomies. The speaker was an oncologist. At the end of his talk, he encouraged the audience to respond. Six young female doctors in the audience, who had previously been diagnosed with breast cancer, stood up one at a time and told their personal stories. Each of those physicians had chosen bilateral mastectomy with immediate reconstruction.

The speaker seemed dumbfounded. The audience was silent. There was no discussion. I left the room with an uncomfortable feeling. There was now no doubt that I was in need of revising my approach to advising women on surgical options.

DECIDING WHICH SURGICAL PROCEDURE IS BEST FOR YOU

No perfect formula exists for discussing these options, but it became clear to me it was time to rethink my preference for breast conservation. My job, I finally concluded, was to present a balanced discussion on treatment options and allow my patients to make their own decisions. My only caveat was that I insisted they avoid a "rush" to mastectomy. Most of my patients are able to decide on their own which surgery is best for them, though there are still a substantial number who find it difficult to make the final decision.

These are the patients who frequently ask, "What would you do if I were your daughter?"

I now have a new approach to answering that question when it comes to such a personal decision. I ask my patients, "Imagine I have twin daughters who both have the exact diagnosis you have. I would discuss options of care with them in the same way I have discussed it with you.

"If, after this discussion, one of the twins decides on BCS, I would give her a hug and tell her she had made a good decision. If the second twin then states she wants a mastectomy, and I am convinced she has given it careful thought, I'd also give her a hug and tell her she'd chosen well."

My job, then, is simply to help my patients make an informed choice. When they look back on their decision a few years later, I want to be certain they feel in their hearts that they chose correctly.

Actual life is never quite as simple as the example of my theoretical twin daughters. So much progress has been made in both lumpectomy and mastectomy, it is not fair for the surgeon to simply leave all the decision-making up to patients. There are situations, in my opinion, where it is incumbent on the surgeon to point out the merits of one approach over another.

A case in point is a woman who has large, pendulous breasts and a cancer as large as two inches in diameter. Certainly, she is a candidate for mastectomy, but in my experience women with such breasts simply do much better with BCS. With these patients we use a team approach. The surgeon does a removal of the cancer with a generous rim of normal tissue. The plastic surgeon then mobilizes and rearranges the breast tissue to create a more youthful appearance. After that, the plastic surgeon performs a reduction on the other side to ensure breast symmetry. The results of this combined procedure are so favorable that most patients tell us they have not looked so good in decades.

A second example goes in the opposite direction. Women with small (A-cup) breasts often do not do well with lumpectomy. Not only is it challenging to get the entire tumor out without changing the shape of the breast, but the subsequent radiation leads to even more shrinkage (see chapter twenty-six). In my opinion, a much better choice for these small-breasted women is bilateral nipple-sparing mastectomy, or NSM (see chapter twenty-five). One advantage of performing mastectomies is that radiation therapy can be avoided, but the primary advantage is cosmetic. Small-breasted women who undergo nipple-sparing mastectomies are usually overjoyed with their new appearance. They are also delighted to be able to wear clothing that was not suitable for them in the past.

I believe we are transitioning to a new standard in treating women with breast cancer. Yes, we are doing more mastectomies, but what we are actually doing is giving women more choices. Some who in the past would have required a mastectomy now have the option to save their breasts.

Hopefully, we are transitioning to a new standard of care where we respect a woman's choice in having one or both breasts removed to treat a cancer that could have been treated equally well with lumpectomy and radiation. Key to the success of this new paradigm is the availability of plastic surgeons who are specially trained and dedicated to the concept of providing newly diagnosed breast cancer patients with a full spectrum of reconstruction options.

A major step forward in our practice occurred when we added an "in-house" plastic surgeon—who happens to be my son, Justin West—to our treatment team. This facilitates treatment planning and provides women with timely answers to complex questions about reconstructive options, which Justin will review in the following two chapters.

WHAT I'D TELL MY DAUGHTER

- Survival is not improved with mastectomy: Survival rates with lumpectomy are equal to survival rates with mastectomy.

- Lumpectomy is my first choice in treating breast cancer when it is technically possible to do it.

- The final decision should always be the patient's.

CHAPTER TWENTY-FIVE

Breast Reconstruction After Mastectomy

by Justin West, MD

For PATIENTS with breast cancer, "mastectomy" is a scary word. For many, it conjures images of loved ones who have been through it, often with disfiguring and dissatisfying results.

The good news is that surgical approaches have significantly evolved. Most patients are ultimately able to achieve results that allow them to fit into a bra and feel good about themselves when they look in a mirror. Others get results that are hard to distinguish from our cosmetic breast surgery patients. In fact, it is not uncommon for patients to tell us that they like the looks of their breasts better after cancer surgery than before.

Comments like these are testimony to the evolution of techniques and devices used for breast reconstruction, and are far and away the most gratifying part of being a plastic surgeon.

BREAST SURGEON VERSUS PLASTIC SURGEON

In Europe it is common to have one surgeon perform both the mastectomy and the reconstruction. In the United States, this practice is rare, which, in my opinion, works to our patient's benefit. The number one goal of any woman with malignancy is to make sure the cancer is removed and never comes back.

The breast surgeon who accepts this responsibility needs to ensure that every effort is made to see that this happens. Although he or she should consider the cosmetic impact, the focus needs to be on effective cancer treatment.

The plastic surgeon's primary goal, on the other hand, is to restore a feminine, aesthetically pleasing breast so that the patient can feel whole. The more aggressive the breast surgeon is with removing diseased tissue, the more difficult it can be for the plastic surgeon to accomplish this.

Though a less aggressive approach by the cancer surgeon can make the reconstruction outcome better, it runs the risk of compromising the patient's ultimate freedom from disease. In my opinion, no one surgeon should be faced with the debate between giving a woman a better cancer surgery or a better cosmetic result. The ideal situation means the breast surgeon and plastic surgeon work together, developing a plan that delivers both a safe cancer removal as well as an excellent aesthetic outcome.

BREAST ANATOMY

Breasts vary widely with regard to size and shape, both from person to person, and even from left to right on the same person. The underlying anatomy, however, is the same. Think of the breast as having several different layers, like an almond Hershey's Kiss. You peel back the top layer of foil and find a mound of chocolate. If you then work your way through the chocolate, toward the bottom you find an almond.

Each layer is connected to but distinct from those around it. The skin, nipple, and areola make up the first layer. Below this is a layer of fat. In patients with lower body weight (competitive swimmers and ballet dancers, for instance), this layer can be quite thin. In heavier patients it's often nearly an inch thick.

Farther down is the breast tissue. This is the structure that a breast surgeon focuses on finding and removing. Breast tissue is white, which distinguishes it from the overlying yellow fat. Below this layer is muscle. Muscle is red and easy to separate from the white breast tissue above it. With rare exceptions, muscle is not removed during a mastectomy.

THE MASTECTOMY

The goal of the mastectomy is to remove all traces of breast tissue to ensure that the cancer is removed and does not recur. To accomplish this, the surgeon must first make an incision through the skin. Where the incision is made depends on the size and shape of the breast and the location of the cancer, but it also takes into account the preference of the patient as well as the plastic surgeon.

The incision goes through the skin and continues down through the yellow fat layer until the white breast tissue is identified. The surgeon then separates the combined layer of skin and fat from the breast tissue, similar to how one separates the skin of an orange from the underlying fruit.

The layers of the breast can be challenging to see and are held together quite firmly. It takes a skilled surgeon to find those layers and carefully separate them to make certain that the vast majority of breast tissue is removed, while causing the least amount of harm to the skin that is left behind.

Once the breast tissue has been separated from the skin all the way around, the tissue is then carefully peeled off the muscle layer. The entire breast is taken out as one piece, which brings the cancer part of the procedure to an end.

Skin-Sparing Versus Nipple-Sparing Mastectomy

There are two ways a mastectomy can be performed: *skin-sparing* or *nipple-sparing*. Both involve removal of all breast tissue. In the skin-sparing approach, the surgeon removes the nipple and areola, as well as some of the breast skin. This is the traditional route to mastectomies.

Nipple-sparing mastectomy is a newer procedure. In this surgery an incision is made in the breast, but the skin, nipple, and areola are all left in place. This technique leads to our best aesthetic outcome because saving all of the skin allows us to create a better breast shape. The nipple that is saved does not have sensation, but it is usually prettier and more natural looking than one that we build (more on nipple reconstruction later).

BREAST RECONSTRUCTION AWARENESS

In a place like Southern California where there are more plastic surgeons than orange trees, it's easy to assume that all patients who are diagnosed with breast cancer are given the opportunity to learn about their breast reconstruction options following lumpectomy or mastectomy.

However, the fact is, across the United States, fewer than 40 percent of patients meet with a plastic surgeon after receiving a diagnosis of breast cancer. The American Society of Plastic Surgeons has made tremendous efforts over the past several years to make sure all patients diagnosed with breast cancer have the opportunity to meet with a plastic surgeon to discuss their options so they can make informed decisions on whether to pursue reconstruction as part of their treatment.

WHO PAYS FOR RECONSTRUCTION?

I am frequently asked by patients if breast reconstruction is covered by insurance or paid out of pocket like a face lift. The Women's Health and Cancer Rights Act was signed into law in 1998 by President Bill Clinton, and mandates that insurance companies must pay for reconstruction. The law also states that surgery for the other breast without cancer is another protected benefit. That being said, not all plastic surgeons accept insurance.

Patients seeking care from doctors who do not accept insurance will have to pay out of pocket. The good news is that most plastic surgeons who perform breast reconstruction as part of their practice do work with insurance plans in one way or another.

GOALS OF RECONSTRUCTION
AFTER MASTECTOMY

I find it helpful for patients to share with me their reconstruction goals. Some patients tell me that they don't mind what they look like out of clothes as long as they can fill out their bras and blouses. Others have much higher expectations, often stating that they hope to look the same or better when their reconstruction is complete.

My goal as a plastic surgeon is to make every effort to see that my patients achieve the goals they share with me. An important part of what I do is to set realistic expectations. Not every patient is able to achieve an outstanding result. Some people have a more challenging anatomy to work with. In others, the nature of the cancer sets them up for a more difficult reconstruction.

Whatever the case may be, I always strive to achieve a result that makes the patient feel whole and feminine. I want them to be able to look in the mirror and feel good about what they see. In my own practice I have seen that the better results we deliver, the more confident our patients tend to be.

WHO IS A CANDIDATE
FOR RECONSTRUCTION?

Unless they are otherwise unhealthy, all patients in our practice are offered the opportunity to have a consultation with a plastic surgeon and learn about their reconstruction options. The majority of these women elect to have some form of breast reconstruction.

Patients frequently ask if advanced age will prevent them from being a candidate. As long as a patient is healthy she can be considered a candidate. The oldest patient I have operated on was a ninety-two-year-old woman who was interested in improving her reconstruction results twenty-five years after her original cancer treatment. She still played racquetball three days a week and was in better shape than some of my fifty-year-old patients. She did very well with her recovery and was back on the court four weeks later.

We do take some precautions: Smokers are required to quit four weeks before and after surgery because of increased complications. Patients with common medical problems such as diabetes, hypertension, and obesity may be candidates for reconstruction but should have their conditions well controlled to reduce their risk of postoperative problems. Women who have had recent heart attacks, strokes, or other serious medical conditions are not considered ideal candidates for breast reconstruction. For these patients an external prosthesis worn in the bra is often the safer choice.

TIMING OF RECONSTRUCTION: IMMEDIATE OR DELAYED

Most patients choose to undergo immediate reconstruction, which means the plastic surgery portion starts as soon as the breast surgeon finishes removing the breast tissue. But women may also delay reconstruction for weeks, months, or years following their cancer surgery.

In some cases, patients initially decide they do not care to have their breasts rebuilt, but years later seek reconstruction because they are tired of not fitting into bras, using prosthetic devices, or seeing in the mirror a daily reminder of what they have been through.

In other cases, the surgeon may suggest that the reconstruction be delayed until the patient has quit smoking or has treated another health concern that could compromise the result.

It is important to note that a patient's right to reconstruction applies no matter how much time passes between the mastectomy and the decision to undergo reconstructive surgery.

TWO STYLES OF RECONSTRUCTION:
IMPLANTS VERSUS FLAPS

Two main options are available for patients who choose breast reconstruction after mastectomy: implants or flaps. Roughly 80 percent of patients in the United States elect to have implant reconstruction. The surgery is faster, and patients get back to their normal lives more quickly. With a high prevalence of breast implants in the United States, many patients are more familiar with this choice, either because they have them or know someone who does.

Although performed less frequently, flap surgery is an excellent option for those who prefer or require it. A flap refers to tissue that a surgeon takes from one part of the body for reconstruction of another. The flaps we use most commonly in breast surgery include the TRAM and DIEP flaps from the belly, and the latissimus flap from the back.

Some patients choose flap surgery because they prefer to avoid implants due to personal or religious reasons. Others end up having flap surgery not because they want to, but because they are not ideal candidates for implants, such as those with a history of breast radiation. Skin that has been radiated does not heal as well, and there is a higher risk of complications when operating on radiated skin. Patients who choose to have an abdominal flap such as a DIEP or TRAM often do so because they like the added benefit of having a flatter belly (similar to, but not the same as, a tummy tuck).

Implant Reconstruction Details

The majority of patients who have reconstruction following mastectomy elect to do so with implants. The best candidates for this method are women with small- to medium-size breasts. Implant surgery is also a good option for patients who are having both breasts removed, as well as those who have already had breast augmentation surgery. Implant-based reconstruction is usually performed in a couple stages.

The first stage involves placing a tissue expander under the muscle. The expander is basically a balloon that we use to create new skin as well as stretch out existing skin that deflates when the breast tissue is removed. A graft material is often used during this first stage to help secure the expander and recreate the anatomy of the lower portion of the breast. Fluid is placed in the expander on the day of surgery, then additional fluid is added over the next four to twelve weeks until the patient reaches the size they prefer to be.

The second stage involves an outpatient procedure during which the expander is removed and a permanent implant is placed. The implant used may be smooth or textured, round or shaped. There are hundreds of options to choose from, and it is up to the plastic surgeon to determine which implant will best fit the patient's goals and body.

During this second procedure additional steps may be performed on the reconstructed breast, such as fat transfer, or placement of additional pieces of graft material to improve the overall result. This second stage is also when the symmetry procedure for the non-cancer breast is performed.

There has been a recent trend in what plastic surgeons are referring to as "direct-to-implant" or "single-stage" surgery. This approach to reconstruction involves skipping the tissue expander and instead placing the permanent implant (the final silicone or saline implant) on the same day as the mastectomy. The benefit to this approach is the potential to be done with both the mastectomy and final reconstruction in one day. Although this is possible, many of the studies on this technique reveal a very high revision rate, with up to 80 percent of these patients having additional surgery to improve the result.

A potential concern with this one-stage approach is that the pressure placed on the breast skin flaps may cause irreversible damage that leads to the need for a larger reconstruction.

When a tissue expander is placed, the surgeon controls how much fluid is placed inside. The more fluid placed, the heavier and fuller the expander gets and the more pressure placed on the delicate breast skin. Too much pressure on the skin means blood will not flow, leading to the loss of some or all of the breast skin. With an expander the plastic surgeon can use clinical judgment to determine how much volume to add without placing the skin at risk.

With the permanent silicone implant there is no controlling the volume. The implant is placed, but no adjustments to the volume can be made later. Many surgeons who use this technique report that to minimize damage to the skin they frequently place implants that are smaller than what would best fit the patient. As a result, they frequently have to go back to the operating room for a second surgery to replace the implants with a more appropriate size after the skin has recovered. I personally prefer two-stage surgery. I think it is safer and more predictable.

Flap Reconstruction Details

All flap surgery involves moving living tissue from one part of the body to another. To keep the tissue alive in the new location, there must be a blood supply to deliver oxygen. We refer to this blood supply as the pedicle. You can think of it as the hose that keeps the rose garden alive.

The TRAM flap is an excellent way to rebuild a breast following a mastectomy. In this procedure the fat is taken from the belly to reconstruct the breast. This is the same fat that is removed during a tummy tuck. This procedure can be done in one of two ways, a pedicle flap or a free flap.

In the pedicle TRAM flap the blood supply is kept intact. In the free flap the blood supply is disconnected. The artery and vein that keep the flap alive are then sewn into a new source around the breast. Because of the very small size of the blood vessels, this procedure is typically performed under a microscope and referred to as microsurgery. A potential downside to the TRAM flap is that the abdominal muscles get damaged, leading to a decrease in core strength. Patients find that it can be more difficult to get out of bed, get out of a car, or get up from a chair as a result of the surgery.

The DIEP flap is like the TRAM flap except that most or all of the muscle is preserved. This means that patients do not see the same decrease in core strength that is observed with the other. When only one flap is used, patients don't experience a big difference in strength between the TRAM and DIEP. However, when two flaps are used the difference can be noticeable. For this reason, we prefer to use the DIEP flaps when reconstructing both breasts.

The other commonly used flap for breast reconstruction is the latissimus flap. Unlike the belly flaps, which rely on available fat to rebuild the breast, in the latissimus flap there is usually very little fat. Instead, this flap is based around the latissimus muscle, which typically involves moving some skin and part of or the whole muscle to the breast. The flap is usually quite thin and doesn't provide the volume needed to build a breast. For this reason, an expander or implant is used. The implant provides the volume, the muscle serves as a protective layer over the implant, and the skin replaces the skin removed during the mastectomy. If a nipple-sparing mastectomy is performed, then a flap is created using only the muscle, since no additional skin will be required.

RECOVERY AFTER RECONSTRUCTION

Implant Reconstruction Recovery

Recovery varies from person to person. I have had some patients who have done so well that they did not require any prescription pain medication following surgery. However, the majority of patients do find that they need narcotic pain medication for the first two to three weeks to handle the discomfort following surgery. Patients are usually allowed to shower two days after surgery, and they can often drive a car by the second week. I tell patients they can move their arms but should not do so excessively. Walking is encouraged as soon as possible (ideally the same day as the surgery), but patients are discouraged from formal exercise or lifting more than ten pounds for the first six weeks.

Flap Reconstruction Recovery

Recovery after flap surgery is usually a longer process, due in part to the fact that an additional part of the body has undergone an operation. Patients who have a flap procedure from the abdomen or back frequently have more discomfort than those who have undergone implant reconstruction. Women are encouraged to walk the same day, but this can be more challenging for those with belly tissue used because the area will be sore and tight for days to weeks following the procedure.

Those having TRAM or DIEP flaps also have to walk bent at the waist for the first five to ten days until some of the tightness of the lower belly relaxes. Like the patients who have implant reconstruction, these women are allowed to shower two days after surgery. Patients may take more than two weeks before they feel comfortable driving, and they may not lift more than ten pounds for the first six weeks.

SYMMETRY PROCEDURES FOR THE BREAST WITHOUT CANCER

The Women's Health and Cancer Rights Act requires insurance companies to cover not only reconstruction for the breast affected by cancer but also any procedure that is done on the opposite breast to achieve symmetry.

Some patients who undergo a one-sided mastectomy with reconstruction will be able to achieve symmetry with the opposite breast without having to do anything to the other side. However, I find that the majority of patients get a better match if a procedure is performed for the breast without cancer.

The symmetry surgery may involve a relatively uncomplicated procedure such as a lift, reduction, or augmentation, or it may involve a prophylactic mastectomy and full reconstruction.

Prophylactic Mastectomy and Reconstruction

Over the past decade there has been an increasing trend for patients to not only choose mastectomy over breast-conserving therapy but also to choose a mastectomy on the breast without cancer. Over half of the patients in our practice who choose mastectomy for their cancer treatment also elect to have a prophylactic mastectomy.

Prophylactic mastectomy has the potential to reduce or eliminate the odds of a patient developing a cancer in the other breast. This is a deeply personal decision that should be made after a thorough consultation with various members of a breast cancer team. I think it is a reasonable option for patients who are good candidates for surgery and have given careful consideration to the decision.

The reconstruction options for patients who choose to have prophylactic mastectomy are the same for those who have a mastectomy on one side. For implant-based reconstruction, performing the same procedure on both sides often results in better symmetry. Women who elect to have flap surgery can also benefit if the same flap procedure is performed on both breasts.

Women interested in TRAM or DIEP flaps must have enough tissue that the belly can be split in half and produce two breasts of an acceptable size. I find that many of our patients in California have enough tissue to build one breast but not two. In case of the latissimus flap, there are two sides to use, so sharing is not an issue.

NIPPLE RECONSTRUCTION

Nipple reconstruction is offered to all patients who have their nipples removed during a skin-sparing mastectomy. Although some patients choose not to have this step performed, most patients in our practice who elect to undergo reconstruction consider this an important step.

In patients who have implant reconstruction this is typically the final procedure they undergo. Some surgeons perform this during the second stage when the expander is removed and the permanent implant is placed. Some surgeons, like myself, prefer to perform the procedure three to six months after the second stage. An easy procedure for the patient, it can be performed either in the office or back in the operating room. There is generally no pain associated with this and therefore no significant recovery period.

In patients who have a flap procedure the nipple can be created at the same time as the flap, or the surgeon may elect to perform this during an additional stage.

The final step in nipple reconstruction is adding color so that the nipple and areola stand out from the rest of the breast skin. In the past, many surgeons did this by taking a small skin graft from the groin since this skin is often close in color to that of the areola. Today, however, it is more common to add the color using tattoos, which some plastic surgeons prefer to perform themselves. Others, including myself, prefer to send patients to professional tattoo artists trained in restorative procedures.

Although the nipple reconstruction and tattooing steps are the easiest parts of the reconstruction, they often have the most impact on the patient. I have seen countless patients come in to see me after their tattoos and tell me that after this step they finally feel like they have breasts again.

WHAT I'D TELL MY DAUGHTER

- If you are considering having a mastectomy, we encourage you to see a plastic surgeon to learn about your reconstruction options.

- If you choose immediate reconstruction, make the appointment with the plastic surgeon as soon as possible after being diagnosed to avoid undesired delays.

CHAPTER TWENTY-SIX

Breast Reconstruction After Lumpectomy

by Justin West, MD

IN MY PRACTICE, I find that most patients are aware that they have options to rebuild their breasts after a mastectomy. However, most women, and many doctors, are surprised to learn that there are also options for reconstruction after a lumpectomy.

The goal of a lumpectomy is to remove the cancer but leave the rest of the breast as normal as possible. Studies have shown that when lumpectomy is combined with radiation therapy, the survival rates for patients can be as good as the rates for patients who choose mastectomy. Because the survival is the same, many patients choose to do the less invasive procedure. The surgery can be done as an outpatient procedure, there is generally less discomfort, and the recovery is usually quicker.

Among patients who choose the lumpectomy option, many make the choice hoping to save as much of their breast as possible. They often express to us that they assume the less-invasive surgery will result in a more normal-looking figure.

This is usually true: Most patients who undergo a lumpectomy and radiation do end up with an aesthetic result that is satisfying. However, long-term follow-up studies indicate that up to 30 percent of patients who choose this procedure are ultimately unhappy with the appearance of their breasts. Because of scarring and radiation, a number of these problems can be difficult to fix. In some instances, we can achieve significant improvement only by performing a mastectomy and then doing a full reconstruction.

It is easier for the patient, and more predictable, when reconstructive procedures are combined with the initial lumpectomy, a concept referred to as "oncoplastic surgery." "Onco" refers to the cancer portion of the procedure; "plastic" indicates the reconstruction option performed by the plastic surgeon.

GOAL OF ONCOPLASTIC SURGERY

The goal of oncoplastic surgery is to create an aesthetically pleasing breast after removal of the tumor by the cancer surgeon. By offering procedures for the breast not affected by cancer, we also strive to deliver breasts that are symmetric in both size and shape.

WHO IS A CANDIDATE?

In our practice all patients are offered the opportunity to meet with one of our plastic surgeons to discuss whether they can benefit from an oncoplastic procedure. Patients who are in good health may be considered for this procedure. Active smokers and patients with poorly controlled medical problems are not ideal candidates.

Large-breasted women who would prefer to have smaller breasts are often excellent candidates for a reduction procedure. Women who like the size of their breasts but not the nipple position or shape may be candidates for a breast lift. Women who prefer to have their breasts larger may be candidates for implant surgery. Others may benefit from fat grafting to help make up for volume that is lost when the cancer is removed.

TIMING

Oncoplastic surgery is best performed at the same time as the breast cancer surgery. This allows the patient to only have to go through surgery and recovery once. The other key benefit is that the surgery can be performed before radiation therapy begins. Non-radiated tissue is easier for the plastic surgeon to shape, and heals with fewer complications.

ONCOPLASTIC BREAST REDUCTION

One of the most common operations performed by plastic surgeons every year in the United States is breast reduction. Patients who elect this procedure typically have a history of problems with neck and back pain, deep bra-strap grooves, and rashes under the breasts. Breast reduction surgery creates breasts that are smaller and lighter, which helps reduce or eliminate symptoms while making breasts that many patients find prettier.

All of our large-breasted patients diagnosed with cancer are given the opportunity to meet with a plastic surgeon to discuss whether a breast reduction might be beneficial. We explain that the reduction will markedly reduce the problems associated with larger, heavier breasts.

A stronger argument for choosing breast reduction in combination with cancer removal is that this often allows the breast surgeon to remove the cancer with a wider rim (margin), hence making it less likely that a second surgery will be required to remove lingering cancer cells. Yet another benefit is that a reduction makes breasts smaller and more compact, which in turn allows better delivery of radiation. With all factors considered, the large-breasted patient has much to gain when lumpectomy is combined with breast reduction.

ONCOPLASTIC BREAST LIFT

Though breast anatomy varies dramatically from patient to patient, and even from left to right side in the same woman, a youthful breast—in theory—has a nipple that is well centered, and most or all of the breast tissue sits above the lower fold of the breast (where the bottom of the breast meets the upper part of the belly).

Over time there is a tendency for nipples to drop to a lower position. A nipple that points straight ahead in a woman's twenties may point straight to the ground in her fifties or sixties. At the same time, the breast tissue typically falls, giving a droopy appearance that bothers many patients.

Breast-lift surgery is a common cosmetic procedure designed to make breasts appear more youthful. Patients who choose this are typically happy with the overall breast size. They like the way they fit into bras and bathing suits. They just don't like the appearance of their breasts without support.

The issue for these patients is that they typically have more skin than breast tissue. One way to explain this is to compare this situation to a woman who ordinarily wears a size six dress and then loses twenty pounds. She either needs a new dress or she has to have the dress tailored to her new body. With a breast lift, the plastic surgeon removes extra skin but saves most or all of the breast tissue. The result is a more youthful appearance, both in and out of clothes.

Breast cancer patients may benefit from combining a breast lift with their lumpectomy. The lumpectomy results in a hollow space. If this space remains unfilled, a depression may result and give the breast an irregular shape—particularly true when radiation therapy is added to surgery. With the breast lift, the plastic surgeon can fill the empty space and potentially protect the breast from developing an irregular shape or contour. Knowing that the plastic surgeon is going to help repair the tissue lost from cancer surgery, breast surgeons often feel more comfortable taking a larger margin. The result is a potentially better cancer surgery as well as an improved appearance.

IMPLANT SURGERY

The impact that lumpectomy surgery has on breast appearance has to do with the size of the cancer as well as the size of the breast. Removing a small cancer in a large breast has little effect on its shape. However, removing a large tumor from a small- or medium-size breast can result in a significant change in appearance.

Breast augmentation with saline or silicone implants is the most commonly performed cosmetic procedure for women in the United States. We are often asked to meet with breast cancer patients to discuss breast implant surgery as part of their lumpectomy procedure.

Many of these patients are women who have previously considered breast augmentation but had not yet pursued it. Others, happy with their breast size and shape, have never considered elective surgery. However, when they learn that the cancer operation may result in a breast that is visibly smaller, they often choose consultation with a plastic surgeon to learn their options.

The procedure that a patient ultimately chooses will depend on both her anatomy and her goals. In some women, the breast with cancer happens to be the smaller one. For these patients one option is to place an implant on the affected side, offering improved symmetry. Other women may opt for implants on both sides, resulting in fuller breasts on both sides. Implants can be placed at the time of the cancer surgery, or—as noted in chapter twenty-five—months to years later. Patients who undergo radiation therapy as part of their treatment need to know that some of the complications associated with breast augmentation are more common in patients who also receive radiation.

Capsular contracture, a process in which a thick scar forms around the breast implant, making the breast feel firm and potentially tender, is one of the long-term problems common to patients with implants, and it is more likely following radiation therapy. While it is not dangerous, patients with capsular contracture often need additional surgery to remove the scar tissue and have new implants placed.

FAT GRAFTING

Another procedure, fat grafting, can benefit some breast cancer patients. In this operation fat is collected from another part of the body using liposuction. The tissue is processed and then placed where it is needed. Plastic surgeons commonly employ this technique to add volume to an aging face, to create more projection for deflated buttocks, or to correct contour irregularities in patients who undergo breast reconstruction after a mastectomy.

A lumpectomy invariably results in tissue loss where the cancer is removed. In many patients, this loss is not visible. But for those with smaller breasts, the loss can be quite obvious. This can be particularly noticeable in low-cut dresses, open blouses, or bathing suits. For some patients the missing volume can be improved by transferring fat from one area to another.

FLAP OPTIONS AFTER LUMPECTOMY

The most challenging scenario for the plastic surgeon is a large tumor in small breasts. This is often best treated with a mastectomy and full reconstruction, resulting in both a better cancer surgery and better aesthetic outcome. But for women who still prefer the lumpectomy approach, the plastic surgeon may have to use a flap procedure.

As with a mastectomy, flap surgery involves using tissue from one part of the body to fix another. As we discussed in chapter twenty-five, three of the most commonly used flaps are those from the abdomen or back. TRAM and DIEP flaps involve removing the excess skin and fat from the lower belly to help rebuild some or all of a breast. This is more or less the same tissue removed during a tummy tuck.

Perhaps more commonly employed during lumpectomy is the latissimus flap, which uses skin and muscle from the back for tissue replacement. It is a very reliable flap, but it often results in a scar that patients would rather avoid.

Flap procedures take significantly longer than other forms of reconstruction and involve new scars outside the breast. For these and other reasons, we often counsel patients with large tumors in small breasts to consider mastectomy, followed by implant reconstruction. The cancer is often better treated this way, and the result is typically superior to what we can achieve with the oncoplastic procedure.

RECOVERY AFTER ONCOPLASTIC SURGERY

Patients frequently ask how the additional surgery I perform as part of an oncoplastic procedure will impact their recovery. Although the reconstruction does add to the surgery time, in my experience it does not significantly impact the recovery.

A lift or reduction on the breast cancer side does not add much discomfort. Of course, a lift, reduction, or implant on the breast without cancer does mean that there are two potential sources of discomfort instead of one.

Most of our patients undergoing oncoplastic procedures do very well, and often stop using prescription pain medication within a week of their operation. Patients are encouraged to walk that same day, but they are usually restricted from resuming full activity for four to six weeks. After forty-eight hours, patients are allowed to shower, and most resume driving within seven to ten days.

WHAT I'D TELL MY DAUGHTER

- Plastic surgeons can be helpful in pre-surgical planning for women who are considering lumpectomy.
- Women with large breasts may benefit from a wider removal of the cancer when a plastic surgeon is involved. A reduction procedure on the uninvolved breast ensures an improved cosmetic result.

SECTION VII

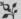

Hope

CHAPTER TWENTY-SEVEN

Better Breast Care for All

I AM OPTIMISTIC about the future of breast care. Yet, despite my optimism, I am concerned there are still unmet challenges that must be addressed.

It's not enough for physicians like me to hope that better governmental decisions will be made in favor of giving women the best possible care. Since this doesn't seem to be happening, doctors need to become organized and force public recognition that poor, even dangerous, decisions are now being made about several breast care issues—such as when mammograms should begin and how often they need to be repeated. As it is, we are seeing an unfortunate trend toward less care . . . sadly, we are going in the wrong direction.

BREAST CARE DOESN'T have to be an orphan among medical systems. Experienced physicians *can* work with dedicated governmental agencies to produce high-value care. I've seen enough success in two other fields—trauma care and organ transplantation—to know there's an effective strategy available for long-term improvement in the quality of care, while at the same time addressing the issue of cost containment.

As described in the Introduction, I have personal experience in the field of trauma care, which started with a fragmented approach when I began my surgical practice in the early 1970s. Back then, if you experienced a serious traumatic injury from an auto accident or fall, you would typically go to the closest emergency room and wait to be seen by the on-call surgeon.

However, in a few cities, such as San Francisco, where I trained, the seriously injured were all taken to a trauma center where an "in-house" team of highly trained experts was immediately available to address their needs. Certain that such a system was preventing many deaths that might occur in an ER, I decided to do a study on trauma deaths in Orange County, where there was no designated trauma center, versus trauma deaths in San Francisco County, where critical accident victims were taken to a single location.

The findings of that study confirmed the value of an organized system of care. Approximately one-third of all deaths in Orange County were judged to be preventable. Among trauma victims treated in San Francisco's designated center, there were no preventable deaths. The study received worldwide attention, reaching the front pages of newspapers in the United States, Europe, and Asia. The medical community was put on notice: There was an urgent need to re-think how best to care for the critically injured.

The surgical community was well aware of these deficiencies. The American College of Surgeons had already appointed a committee to deal with the issue. The Committee on Trauma (COT) established guidelines for optimal trauma care. The remaining challenge was how to get physicians to follow those guidelines, especially at the community level. How do you nudge hospitals and doctors to participate? How do you hold them accountable for their performance?

Just as Medicare had succeeded in making organ transplantation work, another governmental group was given the task of improving the quality of trauma care. The new agency, the Department of Emergency Medical Services (EMS), took on the job of improving trauma care at the local and state levels.

The timing could not have been better. The public was well aware of current deficiencies. The COT had clearly defined optimal care guidelines. The EMS had a mandate from the U.S. government to help physician leaders establish regional systems of care.

In 1979, after a few years of bickering among hospitals and physicians, Orange County became the nation's first organized system of trauma care certified by the county's department of EMS. A limited number of trauma centers were designated. They signed contractual agreements with county officials to provide a team approach to such care on a timely basis, and were held responsible for their performance. Furthermore, on a regular schedule, they were independently reviewed by out-of-state experts.

A study published in a major surgical journal evaluated the first years' experience with the Orange County system, concluding that the problem of preventable deaths was solved. As experience was gained, performance improved and costs were contained.

Care has been similarly streamlined in the field of organ transplantation, greatly benefiting patients and providers alike. Organ transplants started in earnest in the early 1960s when specialty surgeons learned how to transplant new kidneys into patients dying from kidney failure. As time went on, they learned to transplant other organs, such as hearts and livers.

Like so many innovations in medicine, the quality of care was initially inconsistent. In 1971 Medicare agreed to cover the cost of care of kidney failure, including kidney transplantation. Once funding became available, the number of kidney transplant centers expanded rapidly.

In 1984, Congress established a national data-sharing network on kidney transplantation, the Scientific Registry of Transplant Recipients (SRTR). Kidney transplant centers were required to submit a detailed accounting of performance on every patient. The data included a broad spectrum of clinical outcomes on every patient, including key outcome measures such as transplant rejection and post-operative complications.

In 2007, the Centers for Medicare and Medicaid Services (CMS), which paid for transplantation services, took the registry data and used it to certify or decertify existing transplant programs. As a consequence, underperforming programs were eliminated and the quality of established programs was enhanced. Additionally, outcome data was made available to the public on CMS's website, which put pressure on existing programs to compete for the best outcomes of care.

The transplantation story serves as another example of how physicians and governmental agencies can work together to improve the quality of medical care. This evidence-based approach serves as a foundation for the next evolutionary step in care, which is to balance improvements in outcome with cost containment in an effort to produce the best value.

This success can be achieved with breast care patients as well. The task of converting our current disorganized approach into an organized system held accountable for its performance has its own subset of challenges. However, the basic principles remain the same.

First, experienced physicians working at the national level must take the lead in developing optimal care guidelines, as was done for trauma systems. In breast cancer medicine, as opposed to organ transplants or trauma care, there is currently no government agency that has been given the authority to hold providers accountable for their costs and outcomes. Until such an agency is established, care will remain haphazard and costs will continue to rise.

Many of my colleagues believe breast cancer care is so out of control that my proposals are oversimplified and naïve. In their opinion, this field of medicine is just too complex to be organized like the others. I agree that we're faced with challenges, but I disagree that a solution cannot be found. It will take major changes in how we practice. Care must be integrated, and we must be held accountable for how we deal with patients.

In the past few years, we at Breastlink in Orange County, California, have laid a foundation for what can be accomplished as we made our own conversion to a system of care that could be held accountable for both cost and outcome.

Our initial approach was to bring breast imagers, surgeons, and oncologists into one coordinated system with well-established guidelines for care, and standardized methods to audit our results. By coordinating the entire cycle of breast cancer care, from population screening, to diagnosis, to treatment, we have control over every step of the process. We are now able to contract with payers to provide full-service breast care at a fixed or capitated rate. This is an organized approach that has the potential to cut costs and improve outcomes.

Our system could serve as a model for the nation. What's missing is a governmental agency that will work with experienced physicians to make this transition in other communities.

Unfortunately, we are at a tipping point. The government, while so far unresponsive to an organized approach, is desperate for cost-saving solutions. At the moment it is left with two options: Either it employs draconian steps to control costs and accepts the adverse effects on women's health, or it empowers a government agency to work with physicians and together they seek long-term solutions to the breast care challenge.

Where is the media when you need them most?

CHAPTER TWENTY-EIGHT

The Importance of Hope

"Hope is being able to see that there is light despite all of the darkness."

—Desmond Tutu

W HEN A WOMAN receives the call that her biopsy is positive for breast cancer, her life is suddenly turned upside down. "Breast cancer" is an emotionally packed term that conjures up a series of negative thoughts and images. When I call a patient with the bad news, there is usually a moment of silence. I can almost see her expression change and feel what is going on inside her head. After a short pause, there is traditionally an outpouring of questions: "Am I going to survive? How will I raise my children? What do I tell my family?"

My first goal as the physician who makes the call is to take the time to answer all questions in a clear manner, at the same instance pointing out that many issues cannot be explained until further testing is done. It is also imperative to reassure the patient that there is reason for hope.

When the cancer has been caught early and the prognosis is good, hope can be easily restored. However, despite a favorable prognosis, some patients remain skeptical. These patients need added support.

In attempting to restore hope, I tell my patient she will be cared for by a highly experienced team of physicians and support personnel. I emphasize that recent progress has been made in improving the effectiveness of our treatments. In addition, I describe the incredible breakthroughs we've experienced in understanding the basic nature of breast cancer, which will inevitably lead to even more effective treatments.

A major benefit that we offer at our center is a dedicated team of survivors who are committed to restoring confidence in patients who have just been diagnosed with cancer. It is our standard policy to have a breast cancer survivor present when we see the newly diagnosed patient on her first visit to our center. Just having a survivor in the room can be inspiring. The logic is simple: *If she made it, so can I.*

In addition, once we have more information, we assign a second survivor to each patient, someone who is a better match in terms of age and the type of treatment she will be receiving. A good pairing often leads to a long-term supportive relationship.

One of the most essential ingredients in restoring hope is support from family and friends. As one patient put it, "Surrounding yourself with loving family and friends is all it takes to promote and sustain a winning attitude."

Sometimes, though, friends go overboard in trying to help. It is common for acquaintances to share a variety of stories with newly diagnosed breast cancer patients. All too often, these stories are disturbing and misleading. I warn my patients to expect this kind of "help," suggesting that they just thank their friend for sharing the information but ignore the message.

Another warning I give my patients is to avoid the internet. It is filled with confusing information, much of which is inaccurate. I suggest women use it only to search for treatment centers, not actual treatment. If they feel they must do added research, I suggest they stick with the more credible websites such as breastcancer.org, which has accurate information that is easily understood.

For many women, faith in a higher power and the belief that everything in life has a purpose are essential to maintaining a positive attitude. Many patients have shared with me that prayer and the support from their prayer groups were instrumental in restoring and sustaining hope.

Despite our efforts to restore optimism, however, there are times when the outcome of care is less predictable. When a woman is facing a situation in which her chance of survival is poor, the most effective approach to restoring hope is hearing accounts from patients who have faced similar challenges and survived.

Below are stories of two women diagnosed with advanced breast cancer who were told their cases were hopeless and that it was time to start making out their wills. They refused to give up, and their strength and determination allowed them to beat the odds. Their tales are proof of the power of hope.

THE WOMAN WHO WOULDN'T GIVE UP

Susan (not her real name) was forty-one years old when she was diagnosed with stage IV metastatic breast cancer. At the time she had a successful law practice and was the mother of four-year-old twins.

She was found to have twenty-seven separate tumors. Two tumors were in her breast and twenty-five were in her bones. The first oncologist she was sent to told her she had one to two years to live, but only if she underwent aggressive chemotherapy.

Susan was no stranger to breast cancer. Nine years earlier she'd watched her mother die of metastatic breast cancer. She also had a maternal aunt diagnosed with cancer in her early forties.

Interestingly, though they were related, all three women had different types of the disease.

Susan's story highlights the unfortunate reality that even when a woman does everything right, her physician can let her down. Wanting to do everything possible to make certain her children would not witness their mother succumb to the battle with cancer as she had done with her own mother, Susan had BRCA1/2 gene testing immediately after her mother was diagnosed. She was relieved to find out she was negative for that gene. Because of her family history, she did self-exams often and had mammograms every six months.

A year prior to her diagnosis, she felt a lump in her left breast. She went directly to her physician's office, where the physician's assistant ordered a mammogram. The mammogram indicated that the area of concern was completely benign, and an ultrasound was not needed. Susan asked if she could have it biopsied, but she was told a biopsy was not necessary.

It was about this time that she started noticing pains in her legs so severe they would wake her up at night. Initially she was so busy caring for her children and working, she did not seek medical attention.

Several months later, she found a second lump in the same breast. Again she was told not to worry about it. That was when she decided to get a second opinion from a breast surgeon.

The surgeon could easily feel both lumps and a third in her armpit. He had his radiologist biopsy all three lumps and all three showed invasive breast cancer.

Knowing she was facing an uphill battle, Susan decided to do whatever necessary to survive. A PET scan was ordered for the next day. After the scan, the imaging staff told her she needed to see an oncologist, and an appointment had already been scheduled for that evening. The fact that the radiologist was not available to divulge the results of her scan and instead rushed her to see an oncologist only added to her growing anxiety.

It was obvious something serious was occurring and she was desperate for answers. The oncologist and his staff had stayed late that night, awaiting Susan's arrival. She and her husband struggled to remain calm while waiting in the exam room. When the oncologist finally walked in, he seemed uncomfortable with the situation. It was as though he was reluctant to give her the results. Finally, Susan couldn't take it anymore. "Please, fast forward. Is the cancer anywhere else in my body? What did the scan show?"

Although she thought she was prepared for the worst, she was shocked to learn she had advanced stage IV breast cancer. She remembered thinking to herself, "There is no stage V; what I have is the worst-case scenario."

As the initial shock faded, her thoughts turned to her children. Would they suffer the same pain she experienced watching her mother die from metastatic breast cancer?

On the drive home, she and her husband were silent. Just before arriving home, she turned to her husband and said, "I will not go down without a fight."

Her next step was to find the best oncologist she could. When she was seen by Dr. John Link at Breastlink, she was immediately convinced she had found the right place.

Dr. Link explained in extreme detail what could be done to save her life. He noted her tumor fell into the HER2+ category. There was a research trial for a new chemo drug designed to treat HER2+ metastatic breast cancer and she was now a candidate. The research trial offered a new therapy option called TDM1, which was composed of two drugs: Herceptin and Taxotere. Herceptin is an antibody that attaches to protein receptors on the cancer cells. Taxotere is a chemotherapy drug that kills tumor cells. TDM1 has been so effective that study patients often refer to it as the "miracle" drug.

And indeed, Susan's response was dramatic. On the first day of her visit to our center she was in a wheelchair; due to severe bone pain she could not walk. One week after her first treatment the pain improved, and by the end of the month she was able to walk without the aid of a walker.

After her sixth round of treatment, a PET/CT scan showed the metastatic bone tumors had completely disappeared and only one tumor remained, a malignancy located in her left breast. Dr. Link told her more than likely this was the tumor that started it all.

Susan is now a four-year survivor of metastatic breast cancer, and there is no evidence of any malignancy on recent imaging. She understands she may need a lifetime of maintenance therapy with Herceptin, but she is willing to do whatever it takes to watch her children grow up.

A WOMAN'S DETERMINATION WINS AGAIN

Barbara Scott, her real name, was thirty-six when first diagnosed with stage I breast cancer. She underwent a mastectomy only. No reconstruction was done, and she received neither chemotherapy nor radiation.

Her oncologist saw her every six months. She felt completely normal when she went in for her two-year checkup. A few days earlier she'd had a chest X-ray, so the results would be available at the time of her visit.

The X-ray report indicated that her breast cancer had now spread to her lungs. Her oncologist explained that she would be started immediately on chemotherapy. She asked if the chemo would make her cancer go away.

His response sent chills down her spine. In essence, he said it was hopeless. All the chemo could do would be to slow the rate of growth of her metastasis.

With those words, Barbara's hope vanished. She was paralyzed with fear and could not decide what to do next. In desperation she read a book called *The Cancer Survivors and How They Did It* (see Appendix II). The book contained a collection of stories of patients who were told there was no hope—yet they beat the odds and survived. One patient was diagnosed with metastatic breast cancer but was still alive after ten years.

After perusing this story, Barbara's hopelessness disappeared. She decided immediately that if the patient in the book could make it for ten years, she would also become a survivor.

Following her diagnosis, she was given a six-month course of what we would now consider to be substandard therapy. Despite her oncologist's predictions, her next chest X-ray was completely normal.

Twenty-two years have passed since she was told she had metastatic breast cancer. She is now the director of our patient support classes. Over the past two decades, she has inspired hope in hundreds of women who have been diagnosed with advanced breast cancer.

Susan and Barbara were both in desperate situations. Yet patients with a favorable prognosis can also struggle with hopelessness, as is illustrated in Jessica's story.

WHEN FEAR IS YOUR WORST ENEMY

Jessica was fifty-eight when her screening mammogram showed a new density in her left breast. It was marble-sized and looked suspicious. An ultrasound-guided core needle biopsy showed a low-grade invasive ductal cancer. Her tumor markers indicated a favorable prognosis. All she needed was a lumpectomy and radiation. No chemo was called for, but she was advised that taking a five-year course of a hormone-blocking drug would improve her prognosis.

Typically, when a woman gets a favorable report like this, hope is immediately restored. The next question she usually asks is, "How soon can we get started?" Not in Jessica's case. She simply could not accept the fact that she'd even been diagnosed with cancer.

After being told that the next step was a lumpectomy, she shook her head and stated that she was not ready to make a decision.

I explained that "making a decision" was not a problem, since her cancer was slow growing, with a favorable prognosis. Fairly certain of what would happen next, I waited, assuming that when she realized how fortunate she was to have her cancer diagnosed while still at an early stage, her attitude would improve.

I was wrong. She showed no change in mood and still could not accept the fact that she even had the disease. Yet on her third visit Jessica was a different person. She came in with a big smile and was anxious to proceed with surgery.

I asked, "What changed?"

She explained that something very positive had happened on the previous night, when she attended a church dinner. After the meal, the congregation stood and made a big circle, in which they all held hands. A moment of silence was called for, and everyone bowed their heads in prayer.

On closing her eyes, Jessica felt a warm glow that started at the tip of her head and quickly extended to the rest of her body. She knew it was a special sign directed to her, telling her that someone was looking after her. The episode was transformative. Almost immediately, she became optimistic about her prognosis and was anxious to proceed with surgery.

From Jessica's case I learned an important lesson, which I've shared with other patients: Each breast cancer patient has her own pathway to hope. It is important that the care team remain positive, but it is also imperative that they be patient.

We simply cannot rush the process. Sometimes the best approach is to continue offering hugs and to reinforce the fact that we will do everything we can to help restore hope.

Conclusion

IN SPITE OF my optimism, I'm concerned about unmet challenges that must still be addressed.

On the good side, rapid progress is being made in basic scientific research. The secrets of what makes a normal cell transform into a malignant cell are being unlocked at an unprecedented rate. This progress has led to the development of more effective and less toxic cancer drugs. However, we are not completely in the clear yet. These new drugs often come at an outrageous price. It is not unusual for one year's therapy to exceed a price of $100,000. Yet some of these expensive drugs are only effective in extending life by a few months.

Until we find "the cure," it is important to stay focused on today's early detection efforts. New advances in technology, such as 3-D mammography, screening ultrasounds, and screening MRIs, allow us to detect breast cancers in their infancy, when being cured is probable and costly drugs are unnecessary.

Yet early detection has its own subset of challenges. Currently, a large proportion of the population is not participating in routine screenings. It is in this group of patients where breast cancers are detected late and in more advanced stages. Efforts must also be made to lower the cost of screening and improve its accuracy. Until the cure is discovered, we must balance investment in more effective treatments with equal attention to early detection efforts.

As I enter the twilight of my career, I see a new vision for the future. Just as thoracic surgeons were put out of business when a cure was found for tuberculosis, I can imagine a future where the same fate awaits breast surgeons. I can foresee my future employment as a greeter at Walmart. I would be at the front door wearing a white coat and a badge stating: "I am a breast surgeon: Ask Me!" I would direct women with concerns about breast cancer to the aisle containing breast cancer test kits. For those women who tested positive, I would write a prescription for a pill that would destroy any hidden breast cancer cells.

What a life . . . starting with radical mastectomies and ending with writing prescriptions for a cure. It doesn't get any better than that.

Appendix I
Breast Cancer: Risk Assessment

🌿

UNDERSTANDING YOUR RISKS and knowing what to do about them could impact your chances for surviving breast cancer. The process of risk assessment is rapidly evolving, with many ongoing controversies about how it should be performed and who should be tested.

There is, however, a general consensus that we are not doing enough testing. It has been estimated that at least 2 million women in the United States who would benefit from risk assessment are not being tested.

DETERMINING YOUR LIFETIME RISK

Women such as Angelina Jolie with a strong family history of early-onset breast or ovarian cancer can readily be categorized as high risk. At the other end of the spectrum, women with no family history of breast cancer and no history of a doubtful biopsy are at low risk.

The goal is to define risk for women who fall between these ends of the spectrum. The current approach to dividing women into categories is based on the concept of lifetime probability of developing breast cancer. Women who are found to have a lifetime chance of less than 15 percent are classified as low risk. Women with a 15 to 20 percent possibility are categorized as intermediate risk. High-risk women are those with a lifetime chance above 20 percent.

Computer models are used to determine a woman's cancer possibility based on family history and a series of other related issues. The Gail model was one of the first assessment tools that was used to identify women at high risk. It was simple to use and readily available on the web. The problem with the Gail model was that it underestimated a woman's chance of developing breast cancer.

Newer and more accurate models have been developed, but they are more complicated to use. Formal training is required to use the newer models, which are, for the most part, only available in established risk assessment programs. The current goal is to expand the availability of risk assessment programs.

Benefits of Risk Assessment

In addition to the general benefits discussed in previous chapters, there are two practical benefits of risk assessment. The first is to identify women who qualify for MRI screening. The MRI is the most accurate test currently available for screening women for breast cancer. One disadvantage of the MRI is its cost, which can reach $3,000 in some communities.

Insurance companies cover the cost of the MRI if a patient has a greater than 20 percent lifetime chance of developing breast cancer. In the past, the Gail model was used to calculate risk. As noted, the Gail model underestimates the possibilities of cancer, so many high-risk women were denied an MRI.

Newer testing models are now available that are more accurate in determining who is a candidate for an MRI. We have found that a large percentage of women who failed to qualify using the Gail model now qualify when testing is done with newer assessment models such as the Tyrer-Cuzick model, which is more accurate than the Gail model and is my preferred risk assessment tool.

A second practical benefit of risk assessment is determining who is a candidate for genetic testing. The standard approach for determining who qualifies was based on guidelines set by the National Comprehensive Cancer Network, commonly referred to as the NCCN. The guidelines define specific categories of patients who need genetic testing. Insurance companies usually pay for part or all of the cost for patients meeting NCCN guidelines.

NCCN guidelines can be applied to both women who have been diagnosed with breast cancer and women in the general population with family histories of breast cancer. There is a long list of indications for genetic testing for women who have been diagnosed with this type of cancer. The most common reason for testing at our center is for women who were diagnosed with breast cancer by age forty-five or younger, even with no family history of breast cancer.

Separate guidelines exist for women who have never been diagnosed with breast cancer. The most common indicators for testing women with no personal history is a family history of two or more close relatives in the same family who have been similarly diagnosed. The next most common reason is having a first-degree relative (mother, sister, or daughter) who was diagnosed with breast cancer before the age of fifty.

For those who meet the NCCN criteria for testing, a co-payment, typically in the range of $100, is standard. Until recently, the cost of genetic testing was in the range of several thousand dollars. Now the cost of testing has fallen precipitously. Full panel testing (BRCA1/2 and twenty-eight other high-risk genes) can be purchased online for $249 (see chapter eighteen).

HOW TO NAVIGATE THE SYSTEM

One of the biggest problems for women who want to know their personal chance of developing breast cancer is where to go to find out. Until recently, determination of who needs genetic testing was done by a genetic counselor with a master's degree in genetics. With the rapidly expanding volume of women who need testing, there is no way genetic counselors can meet the need. Two recent advances in care are now available to address this issue.

Many mammography centers are doing basic risk screening by taking a family history, which is mentioned in the final mammography report. It is then up to the ordering physician to determine what should be done next in terms of assessment.

The second advance is the rapid development of risk assessment programs. Most large hospitals have such programs. Many physician offices are now doing screenings, and patients who are found to be vulnerable are sent to programs for high-risk patients.

A quick search of the web will usually identify a risk assessment program in many communities, but occasionally resources will be lacking. Another option is to go to NCCN's website, which is open to the public and physicians, for more information.

The site itself is a bit complicated since it deals with multiple aspects of all cancers. However, if you would like to view the information about breast cancer risks and who qualifies for genetic testing on the website, follow these steps:

1. Go to http://www.nccn.org.
2. Register and create a username and password.
3. Click on the NCCN Guidelines tab in the upper left-hand corner.
4. Click on "NCCN Guidelines for Detection, Prevention, and Risk Reduction."
5. Under "Breast Cancer," click on "Genetic/Familial High-Risk Assessment Breast and Ovarian."
6. Click on "NCCN Guidelines (PDF)."
7. Scroll down and look for the page titled "NCCN Guidelines Version—Breast and/or Ovarian Cancer Genetic Assessment."

Appendix II
Support Services

❧

THE GOAL OF Appendix II is to provide women with a broad spectrum of support services that are beyond those available in physician offices. It provides a list of books and websites that can provide accurate medical advice and stories of inspiration to make the cancer journey more endurable.

THE WEB

Although a random or unstructured approach to the web promotes a state of added confusion that we refer to as "Googlitis," there are many websites that provide valuable resources for both the patient and her family.

Websites That Address Breast Care Issues

There is one website that is truly a standout: www.breastcancer.org. This website is accurate and up to date on a remarkably wide spectrum of breast care issues, from treatment to support. Its content is written by physicians who are experts in the field.

The following is a list of other useful and trustworthy websites:

- Breastlink Centers—www.breastlink.com
- National Cancer Institute—www.cancer.gov
- American Cancer Society—www.cancer.org
- Susan G. Komen—ww5.komen.org

- Memorial Sloan Kettering Cancer Center: Integrative Medicine— www.mskcc.org/cancer-care/treatments/symptom-management /integrative-medicine

Websites That Offer Support

- Michelle's Place—https://michellesplace.org
- Living Beyond Breast Cancer (LBBC)—www.lbbc.org/about-lbbc
- LIVESTRONG—www.livestrong.org
- FORCE—Facing Our Risk of Cancer Empowered—www .facingourrisk.org
- Young Survival Coalition: Breast Cancer in Young Women— www.youngsurvival.org/breast-cancer-in-young-women
- Susan G. Komen: Getting the Support You Need—ww5.komen .org/BreastCancer/FindingLocalSourcesofSocialSupport.html
- Breastcancer.org—www.breastcancer.org/treatment/comp_med /types/group

BOOKS

Inspirational

- Hutton, Andrea. *Bald Is Better with Earrings: A Survivor's Guide to Getting Through Breast Cancer.* New York: Harper Wave, 2015.
- Silver, Marc. *Breast Cancer Husband: How to Help Your Wife (and Yourself) During Diagnosis, Treatment, and Beyond.* Emmaus, PA: Rodale Books, 2004.
- Young, Melanie. *Getting Things Off My Chest: A Survivor's Guide to Staying Fearless and Fabulous in the Face of Breast Cancer.* Springville, UT: Cedar Fort, Inc., 2013.
- Port, Elisa. *The New Generation Breast Cancer Book: How to Navigate Your Diagnosis and Treatment Options—and Remain Optimistic—in an Age of Information Overload.* New York: Ballantine Books, 2015.
- Lunden, Joan. *Had I Known: A Memoir of Survival.* New York: HarperCollins, 2015.

- Robach, Amy. *Better: How I Let Go of Control, Held On to Hope, and Found Joy in My Darkest Hour.* New York: Ballantine Books, 2015.
- Roberts, Robin. *From the Heart, Eight Rules to Live By.* New York: Hyperion Books, 2008.
- Canfield, Jack, Mark Victor Hansen, and Mary Olsen Kelly. *Chicken Soup for the Breast Cancer Survivor's Soul: Stories to Inspire, Support, and Heal.* New York: Backlist, LLC—a unit of Chicken Soup of the Soul Publishing, LLC, 2012.
- Feinberg, Margaret. *Fight Back with Joy: Celebrate More. Regret Less. Stare Down Your Greatest Fears.* Brentwood, TN: Worthy Books, 2015.
- Curran, Amy Baker. *Now What? A Patient's Guide to Recovery After Mastectomy.* New York: Demos Health, 2011.
- Lucas, Geralyn. *Then Came Life: Living with Courage, Spirit, and Gratitude After Breast Cancer.* New York: Gotham Books, 2015.
- Lucas, Geralyn. *Why I Wore Lipstick to My Mastectomy.* New York: St. Martin's Press, 2004.
- Glassman, Judith. *The Cancer Survivors and How They Did It.* New York: Doubleday and Company, 1982. (The book that so inspired Barbara, as noted in chapter twenty-eight.)

Medical

- *The Mayo Clinic Breast Cancer Book.* Boston: Da Capo Lifelong Books, 2012.
- Link, John, James Waisman, Nancy Link, with contributor John West. *The Breast Cancer Survival Manual, Fifth Edition: A Step-by-Step Guide for Women with Newly Diagnosed Breast Cancer.* New York: Holt Paperbacks, 2012.
- Love, Susan. *Dr. Susan Love's Breast Book (A Merloyd Lawrence Book), Sixth Edition.* New York: Da Capo Lifelong Books, 2015.
- Mukherjee, Siddhartha. *The Emperor of All Maladies: A Biography of Cancer.* New York: Scribner, 2010.

Appendix III
Finding a Breast Surgeon

T HROUGHOUT THIS BOOK I have frequently suggested that readers contact a breast surgeon for a second opinion. The problem is that many women are not aware of a surgeon with a special interest in breast care. I have a similar problem when one of my patients moves out of state. I usually do not have a personal connection to breast surgeons in the region to which my patients are moving.

My approach to this problem is to go to a website (like www .breastsurgeons.org) that provides a listing of members of the American Society of Breast Surgeons (ASBS). Established in 1995, the society has approximately 3,000 members (including me).

To find a breast surgeon in your area, start at the ASBS home page.

1. Under the "Membership" heading, click on "Member Search."
2. Fill in your city and other requested information and click the option to search by zip code.
3. Then simply enter the radius for the search, and a list of names will be provided. Note: The website does not provide specific information about the surgeons' practices, but most members will have their own websites.

If you are still having problems finding a breast surgeon or are unable to get your questions answered, contact me at beawarefoundation.org.

Bibliography

❧

Dedication

Michelle's Place Breast Cancer Resource Center. "Remembering Michelle." 2014. <https://michellesplace.org/remembering-michelle>

Introduction

Michelle's Place Breast Cancer Resource Center. "About Us." 2014. <https://michellesplace.org/about-us>

West J.G., Trunkey D.D., Lim R.C. "Systems of Trauma Care: A Study of Two Counties," *Arch Surg* 114 (1979): 445-460.

West J.G., Cales R.H., Gazzaniga A.B. "Impact of Regionalization—The Orange County Experience," *Arch Surg* 118 (1983): 740-744.

West J.G., Williams M.J., Trunkey D.D, Wolferth C.C. "Trauma Systems: Current Status—Future Challenges," *JAMA* 259 (1988): 3597-3600.

Chapter 1 | The Controversies That Drive This Book

The Kelly File. "Charles Krauthammer discusses new mammogram study." *Fox News*. February 2014. <http://video.foxnews.com/v/3199477869001/charles-krauthammer-discusses-new-mammogram-study/?#sp=show-clips>

U.S. Preventive Services Task Force. "Draft Recommendation Statement: Breast Cancer: Screening." 2015. <http://www.uspreventiveservicestaskforce.org/Page/Document/UpdateSummaryFinal/breast-cancer-screening>

Erickson M. "Cancer Survivor Creates Campaign to Inform Women About Breast Density." *JDNews*. October 2015. <http://www.jdnews.com/article/20151028/NEWS/151028913>

American Cancer Society. "American Cancer Society Recommendations for Early Breast Cancer Detection in Women Without Breast Symptoms." 2015. <http://www.cancer.org/cancer/breastcancer/moreinformation /breastcancerearlydetection/breast-cancer-early-detection-acs-recs>

Susan G. Komen. "Breast Self-Exam." 2015. <http://ww5.komen.org /BreastCancer/BreastSelfExam.html>

Jolie A. "My Medical Choice." *New York Times*, opinion page. May 14, 2013. <http://www.nytimes.com/2013/05/14/opinion/my-medical-choice.html>

Young R.E. "The History of Breast Cancer Surgery: Halsted's Radical Mastectomy and Beyond." *Australian Student Medical Journal*. 2013. <http://www.amsj.org/archives/3019>

West J.G., Kapoor N.S., Liao S., et al. "Multifocal Breast Cancer in Young Women with Prolonged Contact Between Their Breasts and Their Cellular Phones." *Case Reports in Medicine*. 2013. <http://www.dx.doi .org/10.1155/2013/354682>

Chapter 2 | For Children, Teens, and Women Under Forty

Mayo Clinic Staff. "Breast Biopsy." 2013. <http://www.mayoclinic.org /tests-procedures/breast-biopsy/basics/what-you-can-expect/prc -20020395>

Ronckers C.M., Doody M.M., Lonstein J.E., et al. "Cancer Mortality Among Women Frequently Exposed to Radiographic Exams for Spinal Disorders," *Radiat Res* 174 (2010): 83-90.

De Bruin M.L., Sparidans J., Veer M.B. et al. "Breast Cancer Risk in Female Survivors of Hodgkin's Lymphoma: Lower Risk After Smaller Radiation Volumes," *Am Soc Clin Onc* 27 (2009): 4239-4246.

Chapter 3 | For Women Over Forty

Newman L. "Mammographic Guideline Update: A Nuanced Approach," *ACS Surg News* 11 (December 2015): 1-5.

Tabár L., Vitak B., Chen T., et al. "Swedish Two-County Trial: Impact of Mammographic Screening on Breast Cancer Mortality During 3 Decades," *Radiology* 260 (2011): 658-663.

Coldman A., Phillips N., Wilson C., et al. "Pan-Canadian Study of Mammography Screening and Mortality from Breast Cancer," *Natl Cancer Inst* 106 (2014): 1-7.

Webb M.L., Cady B., Michaelson J.S., et al. "A Failure Analysis of Invasive Breast Cancer: Most Deaths from Disease Occur in Women Not Regularly Screened," *Cancer* 120 (September 2014): 2839-2846.

Saadatmand S., Bretveld R., Siesling S., Tilanus-Linthorst M.M. "Influence of Tumor Stage at Breast Cancer Detection on Survival in Modern Times: Population Based Study in 173,797 Patients," *BMJ* 351 (October 2015). <http://www.bmj.com/content/351/bmj.h4901>

Durning M.V. "Breast Density Notification Laws by State—Interactive Map." *Diagnostic Imaging.* July 2015. <http://www.diagnosticimaging.com /breast-imaging/breast-density-notification-laws-state-interactive-map>

California Legislative Information: SB-1538 Health Care: "Mammograms." 2011–2012. <http://leginfo.legislature.ca.gov/faces/billNavClient .xhtml?bill_id=201120120SB1538>

Friedewald S. M., Rafferty E. A., Rose S.L. "Breast Cancer Screening Using Tomosynthesis in Combination with Digital Mammography," *JAMA* 311 (2014): 2499-2507.

Skaane P., Andriy I., Bandos E., et al. "Two-View Digital Breast Tomosynthesis Screening with Synthetically Reconstructed Projection Images: Comparison with Digital Breast Tomosynthesis with Full-Field Digital Mammographic Images," *Radiology* 271 (June 2014): 655-663.

Kriege M., Brekelmans C.T., Boetes C. et al. "Efficacy of MRI and Mammography for Breast-Cancer Screening in Women with a Familial or Genetic Predisposition," *N Engl J Med* 351 (2004): 427-437.

Chapter 4 | For Women of Childbearing Age: Birth Control, Pregnancy, and Lactation

Planned Parenthood. "Birth Control Pills." 2014. <http://www.plannedparent hood.org/learn/birth-control/birth-control-pill>

Breastcancer.org. "Is There a Link Between Birth Control Pills and Higher Breast Cancer Risk?" August 2014. <http://www.breastcancer.org /research-news/study-questions-birth-control-and-risk>

Wikipedia. "Birth Control." 2015. <https://en.wikipedia.org/wiki/Birth _control>

Bell H., Gudrun P.P., Lynch A., Harle R. "Breast Disorders During Pregnancy and Lactation: the Differential Diagnoses," *J Clin Gyn Obst* 2 (2013): 47-50.

American Cancer Society. "Breast Cancer During Pregnancy." 2014. <http://www.cancer.org/cancer/breastcancer/moreinformation/pregnancy-and-breast-cancer>

Yu J.H., Kim M.J., Cho H., et al. "Breast Diseases During Pregnancy and Lactation," *Obstet Gynecol Sci* 56 (2013): 143-159.

Amant F., Vandenbroucke T., Verheecke M., et al. "Pediatric Outcome After Maternal Cancer Diagnosed During Pregnancy," *N Engl J Med* 373 (November 2015): 1824-1834.

Breastcancer.org. "Treatment for Breast Cancer During Pregnancy." May 2015. <http://www.breastcancer.org/tips/fert_preg_adopt/bc_pregnancy/treatment>

Dunn S. "Diary of a Mastectomy: Giuliana and Bill Rancic." *Glamour Health.* March 2012. <http://www.glamour.com/health-fitness/2012/03/glamour-exclusive-interview-giuliana-rancic-bill-rancic-diary-of-a-mastectomy>

Chapter 5 | For Men

Bing Z., Bai S. "Gynecomastia: An Uncommon but Important Clinical Manifestation for Testicular Tumors." *Open Journal of Pathology.* 2012. <http://file.scirp.org/pdf/OJPathology20120100003_52689298.pdf>

Mayo Clinic Staff. "Diseases and Conditions: Gynecomastia (Enlarged Breasts in Men)." 2012. <http://www.mayoclinic.org/diseases-conditions/gynecomastia/basics/definition/con-20028710>

Carlson H.E. "Approach to the Patient with Gynecomastia," *J Clin Endocrinol Metab* 96 (2011): 15-21.

Chapter 6 | Breast Pain

Kapoor N. "Breast Pain Information." *Breastlink*. 2015. <http://www.breastlink.com/breast-cancer-101/common-breast-problems/breast-pain/>

Gumm R., Cunnick C.G., Mokbel K. "Evidence for the Management of Mastalgia." *Medscape Multispecialty.* 2014. <http://www.medscape.com/viewarticle/477670_5>

Chapter 7 | Abnormal Mammograms: Calcifications and Densities

Nalawade, Y.V. "Evaluation of Breast Calcifications," *Indian J Radiol Imaging.* (November 2009): 282-286.

Weiss, M. "Mammogram Shows New Calcification." (September 2012). <http://www.breastcancer.org/symptoms/testing/faq_screening /calcifications>

American Cancer Society. "Breast Density and Your Mammogram Report." (2015) <http://www.cancer.org/acs/groups/content/@editorial /documents/document/acspc-039989.pdf>

Susan G. Koman. "Core Needle Biopsy." October 2015. <http://ww5.komen .org/BreastCancer/CoreNeedleBiopsy.html>

Mayo Clinic Staff. "Breast Lump: Early Evaluation Is Essential." 2015. <http://www.mayoclinic.org/healthy-lifestyle/womens-health/in -depth/breast-lump/art-20044839?pg=1>

Chapter 8 | Breast Lumps

Young R.E. "The History of Breast Cancer Surgery: Halsted's Radical Mastectomy and Beyond." *Australian Student Medical Journal*. 2013. <http://www.amsj.org/archives/3019>

Mayo Clinic Staff. "Breast Biopsy." 2013. <http://www.mayoclinic .org/tests-procedures/breast-biopsy/basics/what-you-can-expect /prc-20020395>

Breastcancer.org. "Biopsy." October 2015. <http://www.breastcancer.org /symptoms/testing/types/biopsy>

Cafasso J., Kim S. "Fibrocystic Breast Disease." October 2015. http://www .healthline.com/health/fibrocystic-breast-disease#Overview1>

Mayo Clinic Staff. "Diseases and Conditions: Fibroadenoma." May 2014. <http://www.mayoclinic.org/diseases-conditions/fibroadenoma/basics /definition/con-20032223>

Breastcancer.org. "Phyllodes Tumors of the Breast." April 2016. <http://www .breastcancer.org/symptoms/types/phyllodes>

Chapter 9 | Nipple Discharge

WebMD. "Breast and Nipple Discharge: What It Could Mean." September 2011. <http://www.webmd.com/women/guide/breast-nipple-discharge>

Be Aware Foundation. "Nipple Discharge Pictures." July 2015. <http:// www.breastlink.com/breast-cancer-101/common-breast-problems /nipple-discharge/ductgram_papilloma/>

Chapter 10 | Infiltrating Lobular Cancer: The Devil's Cancer

Arpino G., Bardo V.J., Clark G.M., Elledge R.M. "Infiltrating Lobular Cancer of the Breast: Tumor Characteristics and Clinical Outcome," *Breast Cancer Research* 6 (February 2004): 149-156.

Breastcancer.org. "ILC — Invasive Lobular Carcinoma." March 2015. <http://www.breastcancer.org/symptoms/types/ilc>

Mann R.M., Hoogeveen Y.L., Blickman J.G., Boetes C. "MRI Compared to Conventional Diagnostic Work-Up in the Detection and Evaluation of Invasive Lobular Carcinoma of the Breast: A Review of Existing Literature," *Breast Cancer Res and Treat* 107 (January 2008): 1-14.

Mayo Clinic Staff. "Molecular Breast Imaging: Why It's Done." April 2015. <http://www.mayoclinic.org/tests-procedures/molecular-breast-imaging/basics/why-its-done/prc-20129600>

Chapter 11 | Inflammatory Breast Cancer: The Silent Killer

National Cancer Institute. "Inflammatory Breast Cancer." April 2012. <http://www.cancer.gov/types/breast/ibc-fact-sheet>

Szabo L. "Inflammatory Breast Cancers Rare but Often Lethal." *USA Today*. October 17, 2012. <http://www.usatoday.com/story/news/health/2012/10/16/inflammatory-breast-cancer/1617317/>

Dawood S., Merajver S.D., Vermeulen P.B., et al. "International Expert Panel on Inflammatory Breast Cancer: Consensus Statement for Standardized Diagnosis and Treatment," *Ann Oncol* 22 (March 2011): 515-523.

Rueth N.M., Lin H.Y., Bedrosian I. "Underuse of Trimodality Treatment Affects Survival for Patient with Inflammatory Breast Cancer: An Analysis of Treatment and Survival Trends From the National Cancer Database." *Journal Clinical Oncology* June 2014. <http://jco.ascopubs.org/content/early/2014/06/02/JCO.2014.55.1978.abstract>

Clever Home Making. "KOMO News Special Report: Inflammatory Breast Cancer." May 2006. <http://cleverhomemaking.blogspot.com/2009/05/inflammatory-breast-cancer-did-you-know.html>

Chapter 12 | Paget's Disease of the Nipple

National Cancer Institute. "Paget Disease of the Breast." April 2012. <http://www.cancer.gov/types/breast/paget-breast-fact-sheet>

National Organization of Rare Disorders. "Paget's Disease of the Breast."
     2012. <http://rarediseases.org/rare-diseases/pagets-disease-of-the-breast/>
Be Aware Foundation. "Paget's Disease of the Breast My Pictures."
     September 2014. <http://www.breastlink.com/breast-cancer-101/rare
     -breast-cancer-types/pagets-disease>

Chapter 13 | The Breast Self-Exam Controversy

American Cancer Society. "American Cancer Society Recommendations for
     Early Breast Cancer Detection in Women Without Breast Symptoms."
     2015. <http://www.cancer.org/cancer/breastcancer/moreinformation
     /breastcancerearlydetection/breast-cancer-early-detection-acs-recs>
Susan G. Komen. "Breast Self-Exam." 2015. <http://ww5.komen.org/Breast
     Cancer/BreastSelfExam.html>
Thomas D.B., Gao D.L., Ray R.M., et al. "Randomized Trial of Breast Self-
     Examination in Shanghai: Final Results," *J Natl Cancer Inst* 94 (2002):
     1445-1457.
Foster R.S., Costanza M.C. "Breast Self-Examination Practices and Breast
     Cancer Survival," *Cancer* 53 (2008): 999-1005.
Hassan L.M., Mahmoud N., Miller A.B. "Evaluation of Effect of Self-
     Examination and Physical Examination on Breast Cancer," *The Breast*
     24 (2015): 487-490.
Be Aware Foundation. "Breast Self Exam Video." May 2012. <https://www
     .youtube.com/watch?v=0-hUROxC5Kw>
Be Aware Foundation. "Sign Up Reminder." 2012. <http://beawarefoundation
     .org/content/Sign-Up-Reminder.html>
Michelle's Place: Breast Cancer Resource Center. 2016. <https://www
     .michellesplace.org/>

Chapter 14 | "My Mammogram Was Normal, and Now I'm on Chemo"

Strohm E. "Joan Lunden's Fight Against Breast Cancer: I'm a Warrior."
     People Magazine. October 2012. <http://www.people.com/people/article
     /0,,20856573,00.html>
Erickson M. "Cancer Survivor Creates Campaign to Inform Women About
     Breast Density." *JDNews.* October 2015. <http://www.capecodtimes
     .com/article/ZZ/20150930/NEWS/150939987>

Grady D. "New Laws Add a Divisive Component to Breast Screening." *New York Times*, Health section. October 25, 2012. <http://www.nytimes.com/2012/10/25/health/laws-tell-mammogram-clinics-to-address-breast-density.html?_r=0>

Are You Dense Advocacy, Inc. "Giving Women with Dense Breast Tissue Access to Early Detection." 2016. <http://www.areyoudenseadvocacy.org/facts/>

Durning, M.V. "Breast Density Notification Laws by State—Interactive Map," *Diagnostic Imaging*. July 2015. <http://www.diagnosticimaging.com/breast-imaging/breast-density-notification-laws-state-interactive-map>

Kelly M.K., Dean J., Coumlada W.S., et al. "Breast Cancer Detection Using Automated Whole Breast Ultrasound and Mammography in Radiographically Dense Breasts," *Eur Radiol* 20 (March 2010): 734-742.

Berg W.A., Zhang Z., Lehrer D., Jong R.A. "Detection of Breast Cancer with Addition of Annual Screening Ultrasound or a Single Screening MRI to Mammography in Women with Elevated Breast Cancer Risk," *JAMA* 307 (April 2012): 1394-1404.

Schattner E. "Automated Ultrasound Can Improve Breast Cancer Detection in Women With Dense Breasts." *Forbes* Pharma & Healthcare. April 2015. <http://www.forbes.com/sites/elaineschattner/2015/04/07/ge-healthcares-automated-breast-ultrasound-system-abus-improves-cancer-detection-in-dense-breasts/#74a8a8236f4c>

Kriege M., Brekelmans C.T., Boetes C., et al. "Efficacy of MRI and Mammography for Breast-Cancer Screening in Women with a Familial or Genetic Predisposition," *N Engl J Med* 351 (2004): 427-437.

Friedewald S.M., Rafferty E.A., Rose S.L. "Breast Cancer Screening Using Tomosynthesis in Combination with Digital Mammography," *JAMA* 311 (2014): 2499-2507.

Norton R. "3D Mammograms May Improve Breast Cancer Screening: Higher Detection Rates, Fewer False Alarms Seen with Newer Technology, Study Says." *WebMD News Archive*. June 2014. http://www.webmd.com/breast-cancer/news/20140624/3d-mammograms-may-improve-breast-cancer-screening

Skaane P., Dandos A.I., Gullien R. "Comparison of Digital Mammography Alone and Digital Mammography Plus Tomosynthesis in a Population-based Screening Program." *Radiology* 272 (April 2013).

Chapter 15 | Shame on You, Dr. Krauthammer: Why He's Wrong About Mammograms

The Kelly File. "Charles Krauthammer Discusses New Mammogram Study." *Fox News*. February 13, 2014. <http://video.foxnews.com/v /3199477869001/charles-krauthammer-discusses-new-mammogram -study/?#sp=show-clips>

Miller A.B., Wall C., Baines C., et al. "Twenty Five Year Follow-Up for Breast Cancer Incidence and Mortality of the Canadian National Breast Screening Study: Randomized Screening Trial," *British Medical J* 348 (February 2014): g366.

France, L. "ABC's Amy Robach Discovers Cancer After On-Air Mammogram." November 11, 2013. http://www.cnn.com/2013/11/11 /showbiz/celebrity-news-gossip/amy-robach-gma-cancer

Heywang-Köbrunner S.H., Schreer I., Hacker A., et al. "Conclusions for Mammography Screening After 25-Year Follow-Up of the Canadian National Breast Cancer Screening Study (CNBSS)," *Eur Radiol* 26 (February 2016): 342-350.

Kopans D.B. "The Most Recent Breast Cancer Screening Controversy About Whether Mammographic Screening Benefits Women at Any Age: Nonsense and Nonscience," *AJR* 180 (January 2003): 21-26.

Weiss M. "Garbage In, Garbage Out: A Flawed Study Cannot Measure the Value of Mammograms." *Huffington Post*. April 2014. <http:// www.huffingtonpost.com/marisa-weiss-md/garbage-in-garbage-out-a -_b_4824005.html>

Boyd N.F., Jung R.A., Yaffe A.J., et al. "A Critical Appraisal of the Canadian National Breast Cancer Study," *Radiology* 189 (January 1994): 661-663.

Boyd N.F. "The Review of Randomization in the Canadian National Breast Screening Study: Is the Debate Over?" *Canadian Medical Association* 156 (1977): 207-209.

Coldman A., Phillips N., Wilson C., et al. "Pan-Canadian Study of Mammography Screening and Mortality From Breast Cancer," *Natl Cancer Inst* 106 (July 2014): 1-7.

Webb M.L., Cady B., Michaelson J.S., et al. "A Failure Analysis of Invasive Breast Cancer: Most Deaths From Disease Occur in Women Not Regularly Screened," *Cancer* 120 (Sept. 2014): 2839-2846.

Chapter 16 | Mammograms: The Spin Stops Here

Coldman A., Phillips N., Wilson C., et al. "Pan-Canadian Study of Mammography Screening and Mortality from Breast Cancer," *Natl Cancer Inst* 106 (July 2014): 1-7.

Mammography Education, Inc. "A Commentary by F. Lee Tucker, M.D., FCAP., Virginia Biomedical Laboratories, LLC." 2016. <http://www.mammographyed.com/drtabar/default.aspx>

Shapiro S. "Evidence on Screening for Breast Cancer from a Randomized Trial," *Cancer* 39 (June 1977): 2772-2778.

Tabár L., Vitak B., Chen T.H., et al. "Swedish Two-County Trial: Impact of Mammographic Screening on Breast Cancer Mortality During 3 Decades," *Radiology* 260 (September 2011): 658-663.

U.S. Preventive Services Task Force: "Draft Recommendation Statement: Breast Cancer Screening." 2015. <http://www.uspreventiveservices taskforce.org/Page/Document/RecommendationStatementDraft/breast-cancer-screening>

Kopans D.B., Feig S.A. "The Canadian National Breast Screening Study: A Critical Review," *AJR* 161 (1993): 755-760.

Heywang-Köbrunner S.H., Schreer I., Hacker A., et al. "Conclusions for Mammography Screening After 25-Year Follow-Up of the Canadian National Breast Cancer Screening Study (CNBSS)," *Eur Radiol* 26 (May 2015): 1-9.

Toomey A. "Giuliana Rancic Shares Emotional Story About Woman Battling Breast Cancer, Insists We Will Find a Cure." *The Rundown.* October 2014. <http://www.eonline.com/news/589195/giuliana-rancic-shares-emotional-story-about-woman-battling-breast-cancer-insists-we-will-find-a-cure>

Webb M.L., Cady B., Michaelson J.S., et al. "A Failure Analysis of Invasive Breast Cancer: Most Deaths from Disease Occur in Women Not Regularly Screened," *Cancer* 120 (September 2014): 2839-2846.

Konner M. "Watch the Hype: Cancer Treatment Still Has Far to Go." *Wall Street Journal.* March 17, 2016. <http://www.wsj.com/articles/watch-the-hype-cancer-treatment-still-has-far-to-go-1458231884>

Chapter 17 | Your Bra: A No-Phone Zone

Dr. Oz Show. "Why You Should Keep Your Cellphone Out of Your Bra." December 6, 2013. <http://www.doctoroz.com/episode/why-you-should -keep-your-cell-phone-out-your-bra>

Fantz T. "My Daughter's Story of Cell Phone Breast Cancer." *Towards Better Health.* May 2015. <http://mieuxprevenir.blogspot.com/2015/05/my -daughters-story-of-cell-phone-breast.html>

Consumers for Safe Phones. "Apple Warns Customers to Never Use or Carry an iPhone in Your Pocket." May 2012. <http://consumers4safephones .com/apple-warns-customers-to-never-use-or-carry-an-iphone-in-your -pocket/>

Farber A. "Cell Phone Manual Warnings." *It Takes Time.* June 2015. <http:// it-takes-time.com/2015/06/cell-phone-manual-warnings.html>

Federal Communication Commission (FCC). "Radio Frequency Safety." August 1996. <https://www.fcc.gov/encyclopedia/radio-frequency-safety>

Agarwal A., Deepinder F., Sharma R.K., et al. "Effect of Cell Phone Usage on Semen Analysis in Men Attending Infertility Clinic: An Observational Study," *Fertility and Sterility* 89 (January 2008): 124-128.

Adams J.A., Galloway T.S., Mondal D., et al. "Effect of Mobile Telephones on Sperm Quality: A Systematic Review and Meta-Analysis," *Enviorn Int.* September 2011. <http://www.sciencedirect.com/science/article/pii /S0160412014001354>

Procter R.N. "The History of the Discovery of the Cigarette–Lung Cancer Link: Evidentiary Traditions, Corporate Denial, Global Toll," *Tobacco Control* 21 (2012): 87-91.

Ronckers C.M., Land C., Miller J.S., et al. "Cancer Mortality Among Women Frequently Exposed to Radiographic Examinations for Spinal Disorders," *Radiat Res* 174 (2010): 83-90.

Terenziani M., Casalini P., Scaperrotta G. "Occurrence of Breast Cancer After Chest Wall Irradiation for Pediatric Cancer, as Detected by a Multimodal Screening Program," *Int J Radiat Oncol Biol Phys* 85 (January 2013): 35-39.

Gorsky D. "No, Carrying Your Cell Phone in Your Bra Will Not Cause Breast Cancer No Matter What Dr. Oz Says," *Science-Based Medicine.* December 2013. <http://www.sciencebasedmedicine.org/no-carrying -your-cell-phone-in-your-bra-will-not-cause-breast-cancer-no-matter -what-dr-oz-says/>

Centers for Disease Control and Prevention. "History of the Surgeon General's Reports on Smoking and Health." December 2006. <http://www.cdc.gov/tobacco/data_statistics/sgr/history/>

Meier B. "Philip Morris Admits Evidence Shows Smoking Causes Cancer," *New York Times*. October 13, 1999. <http://www.nytimes.com/1999/10/13/us/philip-morris-admits-evidence-shows-smoking-causes-cancer.html>

Consumers for Safe Phones. "FCC's Cell Phone Testing Dummy Is Larger Than 97% of All Cell Phone Users." November 2011. <http://consumers4safephones.com/fccs-cell-phone-testing-dummy-is-larger-than-97-of-all-cell-phone-users/>

EMF Explained Series. "SAR Explained." <http://www.emfexplained.info/?ID=25585>

Noble G. "Wall Street's Cell Phone Litigation Problem." LinkedIn. November 2014. <www.linkedin.com/pulse/20141114012451-22544290-wall-street-s-cell-phone-litigation-problem>

West J.G., Kapoor N.S., Liao S., et al. "Multifocal Breast Cancer in Young Women with Prolonged Contact Between Their Breasts and Their Cellular Phones." *Case Reports in Medicine*. 2013. <http://www.dx.doi.org/10.1155/2013/354682>

Environmental Health Trust. "Cell Phones and Breast Cancer." 2016. http://ehtrust.org/cell-phones-radiation-3/cell-phones-and-breast-cancer/

Knutson R. "Case on Health Risk from Cellphones Is Back in Court." *Wall Street Journal*. November 22, 2015. <http://www.wsj.com/articles/case-on-health-risk-from-cellphones-is-back-in-court-1448235126>

Moskowitz J.M. "National Toxicology Program Finds Cell Phone Radiation Causes Cancer." *Electromagnetic Radiation Safety*. May 2016. <http://www.saferemr.com>

Chapter 18 | Genetic Testing

Color Genomics. "Understanding Your Genetic Risks for Breast and Ovarian Cancer." 2016. <https://getcolor.com/?gclid=CJb70IampMkCFQiVfgodfp4EGA>

King M. C., Levy-Lehad E., Lehad A. "Population-Based Screening for *BRCA1* and *BRCA2*," *JAMA* 312 (September 2014): 1091-1092.

Kriege M., Brekelmans C.T., Boetes C. et al. "Efficacy of MRI and Mammography for Breast-Cancer Screening in Women with a Familial or Genetic Predisposition," *N Engl J Med* 351 (2004): 427-437.

National Human Genome Research Institute. "Genetic Discrimination." July 2014. <http://www.genome.gov/10002077>

Chapter 19 | Beating the Genetic Odds: Exercise, Diet, and Weight Control

Blumenthal J.A., Babyak M.A., Moore K. "Effects of Exercise Training on Older Patients with Major Depression," *Arch Intern Med* 159 (1999): 2349-2356.

Smith R. "Breast Cancer Risk Lower in Women Who Walk 30 Minutes a Day for Years." *The Telegraph*. August 11, 2014. <http://www.telegraph.co.uk/news/health/news/11024200/Breast-cancer-risk-lower-in-women-who-walk-30-minutes-a-day-for-years.html>

Institute of Food Research. "Wheat a Plant That Changed the World." <http://www.allaboutwheat.info/history.html>

Dartmouth-Hitchcock Norris Cotton Cancer Center. "Limiting Carbohydrates Could Reduce Breast Cancer Recurrence in Women with Positive IGF1 Receptor." June 2014. <http://cancer.dartmouth.edu/about_us/newsdetail/70998/>

Panagiotis F., Christopoulos P.M., Michael K. "The Role of the Insulin-Like Growth Factor-1 System in Breast Cancer." *Mol Cancer*. 2015. <http://www.ncbi.nlm.nih.gov/pubmed/25743390>

Gasparro A. "FDA Seeks to Redefine 'Healthy.'" *Wall Street Journal*. May 11, 2016. <http://www.wsj.com/articles/fda-seeks-to-redefine-healthy-1462872601>

Banks S. "The Sugar to Fiber Dietary Ratio." *Thinking About Nutrition*. November 2011. <www.thinkingaboutnutrition.com/2011/11/the-sugar-to-fiber-dietary-ratio/>

Bao Y., Han J., Hu F.B., et al. "Association of Nut Consumption with Total and Cause-Specific Mortality," *N Engl J Med* 369 (November 2013): 2001-2011.

Bianchini F., Kaaks R., Vainio H. "Overweight, Obesity, and Cancer Risk," *Lancet Oncol* 9 (2002): 565-574.

Hitti M. "Pine Nut Oil May Cut Appetite." WebMD. March 2006. <http://www.webmd.com/diet/20060328/pine-nut-oil-cut-appetite>

Chapter 20 | Alcohol, Vitamins, and Hormones: What Helps and What Hurts

Centers for Disease Control and Prevention. "Alcohol and Public Health." October 2015. <http://www.cdc.gov/alcohol/fact-sheets/binge-drinking.htm>

Fuchs C., Meir J., Stampfer M.J., Colditz G.A., et al. "Alcohol Consumption and Mortality Among Women," *New England J Med* 332 (May 1995): 1245-1250.

Park S.Y., Kolonel L.N., Lim U., et al. "Alcohol Consumption and Breast Cancer Risk Among Women from Five Ethnic Groups with Light to Moderate Intakes: The Multiethnic Cohort Study," *Int J Cancer* 134 (2014): 1504-1510.

Romieu I., Scoccianti C., Chajès V., et al. "Alcohol Intake and Breast Cancer in the European Prospective Investigation into Cancer and Nutrition," *Int J Cancer* 137 (2015): 1921-1930.

MedicineNet. "Alcohol and Nutrition: How Alcohol Is Metabolized." March 2014. <http://www.medicinenet.com/alcohol_and_nutrition/page3.htm>

Drayton H. "The Truth About Fat Loss and Alcohol." *Get Healthy.* 2015. <https://gethealthy.education/fat-loss-alcohol/>

Islam T., Ito H., Sueta A. "Alcohol and Dietary Folate Intake and the Risk of Breast Cancer: A Case-Control Study in Japan," *Eur J Cancer Prev* 22 (2013): 358-366.

Peppone L., Rickles A.S., Janelsin M.J., et al. "The Association Between Breast Cancer Prognostic Indicators and Serum 25-OH Vitamin D Levels," *Breast Oncology* 19 (2012): 2590-2599.

Whiteman, H. "High Vitamin D Levels May Increase Breast Cancer Survival." March 2014. <http://www.breastcancer.org/risk/factors/low_vit_d>

Barret-Connor E. "The Estrogen Elixir: A History of Hormone Replacement Therapy in America," *N Engl J Med* 357 (October 2007): 1670-1671.

Chlebowski R.T., Hendrix S.L., Langer R.D., et al. "Influence of Estrogen Plus Progestin on Breast Cancer and Mammography in Healthy Postmenopausal Women," *JAMA* 289 (2003): 3243-3253.

Manson J.E., Chlebowski R.T., Stefanick M.L., et al. "Menopausal Hormone Therapy and Health Outcomes During the Intervention and Extended Post-Stopping Phases of the Women's Health Initiative Randomized Trials," *JAMA* 310 (October 2013): 1353-1368.

Joshi P.A., Goodwin P.J., Khokha R., et al. "Progesterone Exposure and Breast Cancer Risks: Understanding the Biological Roots," *JAMA Oncol* 1 (June 2015): 283-285.

Harvey J.A., Pinkerton J.V., Baracat E.C., et al. "Breast Density Changes in a Randomized Controlled Trial Evaluating Bazedoxifene/Conjugated Estrogens," *Menopause* 20 (February 2013): 138-145.

Chapter 21 | "Why Me?"... Think DDT: The Connection Between Environmental Toxins and Cancer

U.S. Department of Health and Human Services. "Annual Report President's Cancer Panel: Reducing Environmental Cancer Risks: What We Can Do Now?" 2008–2009. <http://deainfo.nci.nih.gov/advisory/pcp/annual Reports/pcp08-09rpt/PCP_Report_08-09_508.pdf>

Herr H.W. "Percivall Pott, the Environment and Cancer." April 2010. <http://onlinelibrary.wiley.com/store/10.1111/j.1464-410X.2011.10487.x/asset /j.1464-410X.2011.10487.x.pdf;jsessionid=0D31C657BDE1E1109594 F14EE1B970ED.f03t02?v=1&t=io7i3bl4&s=c0f63b2b737d39aeceb66 e14a187ca169b724ac0>

Cohen B.A., La Merrill M., Krigbaum N.Y., et al. "DDT Exposure in Utero and Breast Cancer." *J Clin Endocrinol Metab,* 100 (August 2015): 2865-2872.

Carson R. *Silent Spring.* Boston: Houghton Mifflin, 1962.

Ronckers C.M., Land C., Miller J.S., et al. "Cancer Mortality Among Women Frequently Exposed to Radiographic Examinations for Spinal Disorders," *Radiat Res* 174 (2010): 83-90.

Amant F., Vandenbroucke T., Verheecke M., et al. "Pediatric Outcome After Maternal Cancer Diagnosed During Pregnancy," *N Engl J Med* 373 (November 2015): 1824-1834.

Mascarelli A. "BPA Is Still Everywhere, and Mounting Evidence Suggests Harmful Effects." *The Washington Post,* Health and Science section. December 9, 2013. <http://www.washingtonpost.com/national/health -science/bpa-is-still-everywhere-and-mounting-evidence-suggests -harmful-effects/2013/12/06/2ff4a462-5b5d-11e3-a49b-90a0e156254b _story.html>

Dhimolea K., Wadia P.R., Murry T.J., et al. "Prenatal Exposure to BPA Alters the Epigenome of the Rat Mammary Gland and Increases the Propensity to Neoplastic Development." *Environmental Health News.* November

2014. <http://journals.plos.org/plosone/article?id=10.1371/journal.pone.0099800>

Morris J. "Study Spotlights High Breast Cancer Risk for Plastics Workers." *The Center for Public Integrity.* November 2012. <http://www.publicintegrity.org/2012/11/19/11806/study-spotlights-high-breast-cancer-risk-plastics-workers>

Woodruff T.J., Zota A.R., Schwartz J.M. "Environmental Chemicals in Pregnant Women in the United States: NHANES 2003–2004," *Environ Health Perspective* 119 (June 2011): 878-885.

Rudel R.A., Fenton S.E., Ackerman J.M., et al. "Environmental Exposures and Mammary Gland Development," *Environ Health Perspective* 119 (August 2011): 1053-1061.

Websites with information on toxins and the environment:
- Silent Spring Institute: http://www.silentspring.org/about-us
- Breast Cancer Fund: http://www.breastcancerfund.org/about

Chapter 22 | Just Diagnosed: Questions You Might Have

Breastcancer.org. "Your Guide to the Breast Cancer Pathology Report." 2010. <http://www.breastcancer.org/Images/Pathology_Report_Bro_V14_FINAL_tcm8-333315.pdf>

American Joint Committee on Cancer. "Breast Cancer Staging, 7th Edition." 2009. <https://cancerstaging.org/references-tools/quickreferences/Documents/BreastMedium.pdf>

American Cancer Society. "How Is Breast Cancer Staged?" June 2015. <http://www.cancer.org/cancer/breastcancer/detailedguide/breast-cancer-staging>

Breastcancer.org "FDA Approves Using Perjeta Before Surgery to Treat High-Risk HER2-Positive Breast Cancer." October 2013. <http://www.breastcancer.org/research-news/20131004-2>

Link J.M. *The Breast Cancer Survival Manual: A Step-by-Step Guide for Women with Newly Diagnosed Breast Cancer, Fifth Edition.* New York: Henry Holt, 2012.

Cancer Research UK. "Lymphoedema After Breast Cancer Treatment." July 2014. <http://www.cancerresearchuk.org/about-cancer/type/breast-cancer/treatment/lymphoedema-after-breast-cancer-treatment>

Soran A., Ozmen T., McGuire K.P., et al. "The Importance of Detection of Subclinical Lymphedema for the Prevention of Breast Cancer-Related

Clinical Lymphedema After Axillary Lymph Node Dissection; a Prospective Observational Study," *Lymphat Res Biol* 12 (December 2014): 289-294.

Kissin M.W., Rovere G.Q., Easton D., Westbury G. "Risk of Lymphoedema Following the Treatment of Breast Cancer," *British J Surg* 73 (December 2005): 580-584.

National Cancer Institute. "Sentinel Lymph Node Biopsy." August 2011. <http://www.cancer.gov/about-cancer/diagnosis-staging/staging/sentinel-node-biopsy-fact-sheet>

Giuliano A.E., Hunt K.K., Ballman K.V., et al. "Axillary Dissection vs. No Axillary Dissection in Women with Invasive Breast Cancer and Sentinel Node Metastasis: A Randomized Clinical Trial," *JAMA* 305 (2011): 569-575.

American Cancer Society. "Radiation Therapy for Breast Cancer." September 2014. <http://www.cancer.org/cancer/breastcancer/detailedguide/breast-cancer-treating-radiation>

Liu F.F., Shi W., Done S.J. "Identification of a Low-Risk Luminal A Breast Cancer Cohort That May Not Benefit from Breast Radiotherapy," *J Clin Onc* 33 (2015): 2035-2040.

Moran M.S., Schnitt S., Giuliano A.E., et al. "Society of Surgical Oncology–American Society for Radiation Oncology Consensus Guideline on Margins for Breast-Conserving Surgery with Whole-Breast Irradiation in Stages I and II Invasive Breast Cancer," *Inter. J. Rad Onc.* 88 (2014): 543-564.

Margenthaler J.A., Vaughan A. "Breast Conservation Surgery and the Definition of Adequate Margins: More Is Not Better . . . It's Just More," *JAMA Surg* 149 (2014): 1305.

Frangou C. "New Guideline Addresses Acceptable Breast Cancer Margins 'No Ink on Tumor' for Stage I and II Patients; Goal of Reducing Unnecessary Re-Excisions," *General Surgery News* 41:04 April 2014.

Rabinowitz B. "Interdisciplinary Breast Cancer Care: Declaring and Improving the Standard." *CancerNetwork*. September 2004. <http://www.cancernetwork.com/review-article/interdisciplinary-breast-cancer-care-declaring-and-improving-standard-0>

Harness J.K., Bartlett R.H., Saran P.A., et al. "Developing a Comprehensive Breast Center," *Am J Surg* 53 (1987): 419-423.

Pal S. "Preoperative Breast MRI: Does Higher Sensitivity Equal Better Outcomes?" *ASCO Post* 5 (June 2014): 1-4.

BreastCancerTrials.org. "Learn About Breast Cancer Trials." <https://www
.breastcancertrials.org/bct_nation/home.seam>

Chapter 23 | Who Needs a Second Opinion—and Why?

Perkins C., Balma D., Garcia R. "Why Current Breast Pathology Practices Must Be Evaluated: A Susan G. Komen for the Cure White Paper," *Breast J* 5 (June 2006): 443-447.

Elmore J.G., Longton G.M., Carney P.A., et al. "Diagnostic Concordance Among Pathologists Interpreting Breast Biopsy Specimens," *JAMA* 313 (March 2015): 1122-1132.

Borowsky A., Esserman L. "When the Gold Standard Loses Its Luster, Perhaps It Is Time to Change Nomenclature." *Ann Int Med.* March 2016. <http://annals.org/article.aspx?articleid=2504523>

Page D.L. "Why I Became a Surgical Pathologist with Interest in Breast Disease," *J Clin Pathol* 60 (March 2007): 251-252.

Dupont W.D., Page D.L. "Risk Factors for Breast Cancer in Women with Proliferative Breast Disease," *N Engl J Med* 312 (1985): 146-151.

Payne V.L., Singh H., Meyer A.N., et al. "Patient-Initiated Second Opinions: Systematic Review of Characteristics and Impact on Diagnosis, Treatment, and Satisfaction," *Mayo Clin Proc* 85 (May 2014): 687-696.

Vaughn D. "Patients in Rural Areas Face Barriers to Treatment." *Cure.* August 2015. <http://www.curetoday.com/publications/cure/2015 /summer-2015/a-country-mile>

Chapter 24 | Mastectomy Versus Lumpectomy

Gutwein L.G., Ang D.N., Liu H., et al. "Utilization of Minimally Invasive Breast Biopsy for the Evaluation of Suspicious Breast Lesions," *Am J Surg* 202 (August 2011): 127-132.

Grady D. "Study of Breast Biopsies Finds Surgery Used Too Extensively." *New York Times.* February 2011. <http://www.nytimes.com/2011/02/19 /health/19cancer.html>

Lakhtakia R. "A Brief History of Breast Cancer." *Sultan Qaboos Univ Med J* 14 (May 2014): 166-169.

Smith C.M. "Origin and Uses of *Primum Non Nocere*—Above All, Do No Harm!," *Clin Pharmacol* 45 (2005): 371-377.

Young R.E. "The History of Breast Cancer Surgery: Halsted's Radical Mastectomy and Beyond." *Australian Student Medical Journal.* 2013. <http://www.amsj.org/archives/3019>

Veronesi U., Cascinelli N., Mariani L., et al. "Twenty-Year Follow-Up of a Randomized Study Comparing Breast-Conserving Surgery with Radical Mastectomy for Early Breast Cancer," *N Engl J Med* 347 (October 2002): 1227-1232.

Fisher B., Anderson S., Bryant J., et al. "Twenty-Year Follow-Up of a Randomized Trial Comparing Total Mastectomy, Lumpectomy, and Lumpectomy Plus Irradiation for the Treatment of Invasive Breast Cancer," *N Engl J Med* 17 (October 2002): 1233-1241.

American Society of Clinical Oncology (ASCO). George W. Crile, Jr., MD, and Umberto Veronesi, MD. <https://www.asco.org/about-asco/asco-overview/society-history/asco50/george-w-crile-jr-md-and-umberto-veronesi-md>

Travis K. "Bernard Fisher Reflects on a Half-Century's Worth of Breast Cancer Research," *J Natl Cancer Inst* 97 (November 2005): 1636-1637.

Silverstein M.J., Savalia N., Khan S., Ryan J. "Extreme Oncoplasty: Breast Conservation for Patients Who Need Mastectomy," *The Breast J* 21 (February 2015): 52-59.

Currie A., Chong K., Davis G.L. "Using Therapeutic Mammoplasty to Extend the Role of Breast-Conserving Surgery in Women with Larger or Ptotic Breasts," *Ann R Coll Surg Engl* 95 (2013): 192-195.

Chapter 25 | Breast Reconstruction After Mastectomy

Spear S.L., Hannan C.M., Willey S.C., Cocilovo C. "Nipple-Sparing Mastectomy," *Plast. Reconstr Surg* 123 (2009): 1665-1673.

American Cancer Society. "Women's Health and Cancer Rights Act." January 2011. <http://www.cancer.org/treatment/findingandpayingfortreatment/understandinghealthinsurance/womens-health-and-cancer-rights-act>

Alderman A.K., Hawley S.T., Waljee J., et al. "Understanding the Impact of Breast Reconstruction on the Surgical Decision-Making Process for Breast Cancer," *Cancer* 112 (February 2008): 489-494.

Breastcancer.org. "Mastectomy vs. Lumpectomy." November 2015. <www.breastcancer.org/treatment/surgery/mast_vs_lump>

American Society of Plastic Surgeons. "Fat Grafting Techniques of Breast Reconstruction Are Commonly Used by U.S. Plastic Surgeons." 2013.

<http://www.plasticsurgery.org/news/2013/fat-grafting-for-breast
-reconstruction-commonly-used.html>

Yoon J.H., Kim M.J., Kim E., et al. "Imaging Surveillance of Patients with Breast Cancer After Primary Treatment: Current Recommendations," *Kor J Rad* 16 (March 2015): 219-228.

Chapter 26 | Breast Reconstruction After Lumpectomy

Clough K.B., Cuminet J., Fitoussi A., et al. "Cosmetic Sequelae After Conservation Treatment for Breast Cancer: Classification and Results of Surgical Correction," *Annals of Plastic Surgery* 45 (November 1998): 471-481.

Spear S.L., Davison S.P. "New Trends in Reduction and Mastopexy," *Semin Plast Surg* 18 (August 2004): 255-260.

American Society of Plastic Surgeons. "Fat Grafting Techniques of Breast Reconstruction Are Commonly Used by U.S. Plastic Surgeons." 2013. <http://www.plasticsurgery.org/news/2013/fat-grafting-for-breast
-reconstruction-commonly-used.html>

Chapter 27 | Better Breast Care for All

Rettig R.A. "Origins of the Medicare Kidney Disease Entitlement: The Social Security Amendments of 1972." *The National Academies Press, Biomedical Politics.* 1991. <http://www.nap.edu/read/1793/chapter/6>

Cameron A.M., Sullivan B.E. "Regulatory Oversight in Transplantation: There and Back Again," *JAMA Surg* 148 (November 2013): 997-998.

Levy R. "CMS Issues Regulations for Kidney Transplant Programs," *Dialysis & Transplantation* 36 (June 2007): 324-329.

West J.G., Williams M.J., Trunkey D.D., Wolferth C.C. "Trauma Systems: Current Status— Future Challenges," *JAMA* 259 (1988): 3597-3600.

American College of Surgeons: Committee on Trauma. "Resources for Optimal Care of the Injured Patient." 2014. <http://www.facs.org/media
/press%20releases/2014/trauma1014>

Shah, M. "The Formation of the Emergency Medical Services System," *Am J Public Health* 96 (2006 March): 414-423.

Porter M.E., Teisberg E.O. "Redefining Health Care: Creating Value-Based Competition on Results." *Harvard Business Review Press.* June 2006.

Chapter 28 | The Importance of Hope

Watson S. "Experimental Breast Cancer Drug Combo Generates Excitement."
Harvard Health Publications. June 2012. <http://www.health.harvard.edu/blog/experimental-breast-cancer-drug-combo-generates-excitement-201206154891>

Glossary

A

abscess: A focal collection of pus in the breast.

alcohol equivalence: The amount of alcohol found in a standard drink. There is an equivalent amount of alcohol in each of the following:

- A 12-ounce bottle or can of a typical beer (5 percent alcohol)
- A 5-ounce glass of wine (12 percent alcohol)
- A 1.4-ounce shot of a typical (80 proof) liquor

alpha-fetoprotein (AFP): A protein in the blood that can be elevated in certain types of testicular cancers. Measurements of blood levels of AFP are done to evaluate breast lumps in males.

alternative medicine: Any type of medical practice that is put forward as having healing effects but is not based on generally accepted scientific studies (see also **complementary medicine**).

areola: The pigmented area surrounding the nipple.

aspiration: The removal of fluid with a needle attached to a syringe. Most commonly done on breast cysts but also used to remove pus from an abscess.

atypia: A term used by pathologists to describe a structural abnormality in a cell.

atypical ductal hyperplasia (ADH): A benign condition in which cells from the breast ducts look abnormal under the microscope. ADH is associated with an increased risk of developing breast cancer.

atypical lobular hyperplasia (ALH): A condition in which cells from the breast lobules, or milk-producing glands, appear abnormal under the microscope. It is a predictor of an increased risk of developing breast cancer.

axilla: The area commonly referred to as the armpit, which contains the axillary lymph nodes.

axillary lymph nodes: Lymph nodes that filter lymphatic fluid that drains from the breast.

B

benign: Non-cancerous. A benign tumor cannot invade surrounding tissue or spread to other parts of the body.

beta hCG: A hormone in the blood that can be elevated in certain types of testicular cancers.

binge drinking: The practice of consuming large quantities of alcohol in a single session, usually defined as five or more drinks at one time for a man, or four or more drinks at one time for a woman.

bioidentical hormones: Hormones that are identical (on a molecular level) to the normal hormones made in the body.

BI-RADS: A schema for putting the findings of mammograms into a small number of well-defined categories.

blind aspiration biopsy: Needle aspiration of the breast performed when there is an area of clinical concern in the breast, but it cannot be seen on the mammogram or on ultrasound.

BPA (bisphenol A): An industrial chemical that has been used to make certain plastics and resins since the 1960s. It is commonly found in plastic water bottles and the lining of tin cans. Elevated levels of BPA have been shown to cause breast cancer in laboratory animals.

BRCA mutation: BRCA1 and BRCA2 are both DNA repair genes. Each individual inherits one BRCA1 gene and one BRCA2 gene from each parent. If a damaged (mutated) gene is inherited from either parent, the risk of developing breast or ovarian cancer is markedly increased.

breast augmentation: This surgery involves increasing a patient's breast size by using breast implants or fat grafting.

breast-conserving surgery (BCS): Removal of the cancer (lumpectomy), but maintaining the shape of the breast. It is usually followed by radiation therapy.

breast lift: A procedure that involves reshaping a patient's breasts and moving the nipples into a more youthful position.

breast reduction: A procedure to reduce the size of the breast and to give it a more youthful contour.

breast self-examination (BSE): A method of looking and feeling to detect a change in the appearance or the texture of the breasts.

C

calcifications: Deposits of calcium that appear white on the mammogram. Most calcifications are not associated with a cancer, but certain patterns formed by the calcifications may indicate the need for a biopsy.

callback: A phone call or letter stating that there were areas on a mammogram that need additional evaluation.

chemotherapy: The treatment of cancer with chemicals that have a toxic effect on breast cancer cells. It is commonly given intravenously (i.e., injected into the veins). The medical oncologist makes the determination of what chemo is best suited for an individual cancer patient.

complementary medicine: A range of therapies that are used in addition to standard medical therapies to promote healing and wellness. These may include acupuncture, herbal medicine, and biofeedback.

core needle biopsy: A type of biopsy using a hollow needle to obtain tissue samples from abnormal areas in the breast.

cyst: A fluid-filled sac in the breast. Cysts are almost always benign (non-cancerous).

cystosarcoma phyllodes: A rare breast tumor that typically occurs in young women. Most are curable with surgical removal. Care must be taken to ensure all of the tumor is removed because if any tumor is left in the breast, recurrence rates are high.

D

DCIS (ductal carcinoma in situ): A type of cancer that is confined to the milk ducts. It is also referred to as stage 0 pre-invasive breast cancer.

DDT: A synthetic poison that was used in an attempt to eradicate malaria-carrying mosquitoes and other potentially dangerous insects. High levels of DDT can persist in the body for years and evidence suggests that high blood levels of DDT can increase a woman's risk of developing breast cancer.

density: Women with dense breasts have an increased proportion of glandular and fibrous tissue as compared to women with fatty breasts. Density is a risk factor for developing breast cancer, and it makes cancer detection more challenging.

diagnostic mammogram: An X-ray of the breast that is designed to evaluate a breast problem (i.e., a breast lump, nipple discharge, or the abnormal findings on a screening mammogram).

DIEP flap: This procedure involves moving the fatty tissue from the lower part of the belly up to the chest to recreate a breast after a mastectomy. The rectus muscles (the "six pack" of the abdomen) are spared to preserve core strength.

Duavee: A new combination drug that includes an estrogen and a drug (bazedoxifene) that blocks estrogen from reaching certain cells in the uterine lining and protects against overgrowth of uterine tissue. In studies, its use as long-term hormone replacement in menopausal women with an intact uterus has been proven safe in terms of both uterine and breast cancer risk.

ductogram: A procedure to outline the structure of a breast duct. A fine tube is placed in the draining duct and a small amount of contrast is injected. The anatomy of the duct is visualized on a subsequent mammogram.

ducts: Breast ducts (or milk ducts) are simply tubes that transport milk from the lobules that produce the milk to the nipple. Most cancers start in the lining of the breast ducts.

E

eczema: A skin condition in which patches of skin become rough and inflamed. Eczema may be associated with itching and bleeding from the skin. Paget's disease of the nipple is often confused with eczema.

EMS: Emergency Medical Services is a system of coordinated response and care for medical emergencies involving transportation and delivery to the appropriate care center, such as a trauma center, in the case of accident victims.

EPA: The Environmental Protection Agency is a governmental agency with jurisdiction over existing chemicals and chemicals under development that can affect the environment.

F

false positive/false negative breast biopsies: A **false positive** is a suspicious area on the mammogram that proves to be negative (noncancerous) on biopsy. A **false negative** is a biopsy of an area of concern on the mammogram or ultrasound that comes back negative when in fact a cancer was present but missed on the biopsy.

familial breast cancer: A history of women who have family members on either side of the family with breast or ovarian cancer.

FCC: The Federal Communications Commission (FCC) is an independent agency of the United States government that is responsible for regulating interstate communications by radio, television, wire, satellite, and cable. The FCC provides the public with information on cell phone safety.

FDA: The Food and Drug Administration is responsible for protecting public health by assuring the safety, efficacy, and security of human and veterinary drugs, biological products, medical devices, our nation's food supply, cosmetics, and products that emit radiation.

fibroadenoma: A solid, non-cancerous breast tumor that occurs most commonly in adolescent girls and women under the age of thirty.

frozen section: A procedure performed when the surgeon wants an immediate answer as to whether breast tissue is benign or malignant. The excised tissue is quickly frozen, thinly sliced, and reviewed under the microscope.

G

Gail model: A computerized risk assessment tool that is available to the public online. The Gail model is simple to use. However, it asks only a short list of questions and often underestimates risk (see Appendix I).

genetic counselor: An individual who has completed a master's degree program in genetic counseling. The counselor evaluates an individual's risk of developing cancer and makes recommendations on the need for genetic testing.

gynecomastia: A swelling or enlargement of breast tissue that occurs in men and boys and is caused by an imbalance of hormones. It can affect one or both breasts.

H

Herceptin (brand name for trastuzumab): An antibody that is designed to target the HER2 protein on the surface of some cancer cells.

hereditary breast cancer: Breast cancers that occur in individuals who have inherited a high-risk gene mutation from one of their parents.

HER2 (human epidermal growth factor 2): A protein involved in cell growth that is present on the surface of about 20 percent of all breast cancers. Women who test positive for the HER2 protein are treated with Herceptin along with chemotherapy.

high-risk biopsy: A term describing breast biopsies that are not cancer but put a woman at increased risk of developing a future breast cancer. The most common high-risk biopsies are atypical ductal hyperplasia (ADH), atypical lobular hyperplasia (ALH), and lobular carcinoma in situ (LCIS).

hormone (endocrine) disruptors: Chemicals that, at certain doses, can interfere with a woman's normal hormones. This can lead to an increase in the risk of developing a future breast cancer.

hormone receptors: Proteins on the surface of cancer cells that influence growth. The most commonly measured receptors are for estrogen and progesterone. Cancer cells that are positive for the estrogen receptor tend to be sensitive to hormone medications such as tamoxifen.

hyperplasia: A term used by the pathologist to describe an abnormal pattern of excessive growth of normal-appearing cells. Hyperplasia is not a high-risk lesion, but it should be considered a variant of normal (see **atypia**).

I

immediate versus delayed reconstruction: Immediate reconstruction of the breast is performed the same day as the mastectomy. **Delayed reconstruction** can be performed weeks to years after the mastectomy. Health insurance programs will cover both forms.

implant: A device used to augment the size or shape of the breast. It can be filled with saline or silicone.

in situ: Refers to breast cancers that have not invaded into surrounding tissue. Ductal carcinomas in situ stay in the breast ducts and lobular carcinomas in situ stay in the lobules.

invasive ductal cancers (or infiltrating ductal carcinoma): Tumors that arise in the breast ducts and extend into surrounding tissue.

invasive lobular cancers (or infiltrating lobular carcinomas): Cancers that arise in lobules or milk-producing glands and extend into the surrounding tissue.

L

lactation: Refers to both the time period during which the breasts produce milk and the process of breast-feeding.

latissimus flap: This procedure involves moving the large muscle (and often skin) from the back to the chest to help rebuild a breast following a mastectomy.

lobular carcinoma in situ (LCIS): A condition in which high-risk cells have proliferated within the breast lobules. LCIS is a risk factor for the development of breast cancer.

lobules: Breast lobules are small sacs at the end of the ducts that produce milk, which is then transported by the breast ducts to the nipple.

locally advanced breast cancer: A cancer large enough to distort the shape of the breast. It is often associated with invasion of the skin or muscle. There may be involvement of the axillary lymph nodes.

local recurrence: A cancer recurring in the breast following a lumpectomy or in the chest wall following a mastectomy.

lumpectomy: Removal of a breast cancer while attempting to maintain the shape of the breast. It is often followed by radiation therapy.

lymphedema: A condition of chronic tissue swelling associated with an abnormal collection of high-protein fluid just beneath the skin. It most commonly occurs in the arms following removal of axillary lymph nodes.

Lymphedema Index (L-Dex): A method to aid in the clinical assessment of early lymphedema of the arm.

lymph nodes: Bean-shaped organs that filter the fluid in the lymphatic system. Positive lymph nodes in the axilla (armpit) are often the first indicator that cancer cells have spread beyond the breast.

M

malignant calcifications: Calcifications on the mammogram that are judged to be suspicious for breast cancer by the radiologist.

malignant tumors: Tumors made up of cells that are growing out of control. These cells can invade into the nearby tissue and spread to other parts of the body.

mammogram: An X-ray image of the breast. A screening mammogram is for women with no symptoms. A diagnostic mammogram focuses on an area of clinical concern such as a lump.

mammographer: A radiologist who specializes in breast imaging, including mammograms, ultrasound, and MRIs.

margin: The distance between the cancer and edge of the lumpectomy or mastectomy specimen. It is a microscopic measurement made by the pathologist. A positive margin means the tumor has extended to the edge of the specimen, and usually requires a second surgery to "clear" the margin.

mastectomy: There are six types:

1. **Simple mastectomy:** Removal of entire breast, but no other structures.
2. **Modified radical mastectomy:** Removal of entire breast and underarm lymph nodes.
3. **Radical mastectomy:** Removal of entire breast and underlying chest muscles (pectoralis major and minor muscles).
4. **Nipple-sparing mastectomy:** Removal of entire breast with preservation of all skin including the nipple and surrounding areola.
5. **Skin-sparing mastectomy:** Removal of entire breast with preservation of all skin with the exception of the nipple and surrounding areola.
6. **Partial mastectomy or lumpectomy:** Removal of part of the breast usually followed by radiation therapy when performed for a malignancy.

mastitis: An infection or inflammation of the breast most typically causing redness, pain, and warmth. Mastitis most commonly affects women who are breast-feeding. The cause is usually a "blocked duct" but can be associated with a bacterial infection. Non-lactating women can also develop mastitis.

medical oncologist: The oncologist is the member of the multidisciplinary treatment team that focuses on the medical treatment of breast cancers. It is the medical oncologist who manages chemotherapy and hormone-blocking cancer treatments.

metastatic breast cancer: Breast cancer that has spread beyond the breast to other organs in the body—most commonly, the bones, liver, and lungs.

milk cyst (or galactocele): A breast cyst that occurs during the period of lactation. Cysts that cause pain or tenderness are usually aspirated, but asymptomatic milk cysts often resolve without treatment.

MRI: Magnetic resonance imaging is a technique that uses a magnetic field and radio waves to create detailed images of the organs and tissues within the body. The breast MRI is the single most accurate tool in detecting small cancers missed on the mammogram.

mutation: A permanent alteration in the structure of a gene. Only a small percentage of mutations result in an increased risk of developing breast cancer.

N

needle biopsy of the breast: There are two types:

1. **Fine needle biopsy:** A small needle is used to extract cells from a breast lump that can be looked at under the microscope to determine if cancer cells are present.

2. **Core needle biopsy:** A larger needle is used to take a core sample of tissue from an area of concern in the breast. The core is approximately the diameter of the lead in a pencil and provides additional information on the behavior of malignancies.

neoadjuvant therapy: The process of giving medical therapy before surgery rather than after surgery. The therapy can be chemo with or without Herceptin, or it can be hormone-blocking therapy.

nipple areolar complex: Includes the nipple and surrounding areola or pigmented area surrounding the nipple.

nipple marker: A small sticky disc placed on the nipple at the time of the mammogram to help the mammographer orient the nipple in relation to other structures of the breast (also used when performing a chest X-ray to avoid confusing the nipple shadow with a possible spot on the lung).

O

oncoplastic surgery: These procedures involve using a plastic surgery procedure as part of a breast cancer treatment. For example, a large-breasted patient can combine a lumpectomy with a breast reduction surgery. The patient potentially benefits from both a better cancer surgery (because a wider margin is often taken) as well as an alleviation of the problems associated with heavy breasts.

open surgical biopsy: The removal of breast tissue through an incision in the skin. This is typically done by a surgeon in the operating room as an outpatient procedure.

organ transplant center: A hospital that specializes in the transplantation of organs such as kidney, heart, or liver from a donor (living or dead) with a healthy organ to a patient with a diseased organ.

P

panel testing: In addition to testing for the BRCA1 and BRCA2 mutations, panel testing includes testing for other high-risk gene mutations that are associated with an increased risk of developing breast and ovarian cancer.

papilloma: A papilloma is a small wart-like growth that starts in the lining of a breast duct. They are the most common cause of spontaneous nipple discharge. They are benign and are usually surgically removed when associated with spontaneous nipple discharge.

pathologist: A physician who makes the diagnosis of diseases by examining tissue, cells, and blood samples. The pathologist examines tissue biopsy specimens to make a tissue diagnosis and evaluates mastectomy, lumpectomy, and lymph node specimens to determine extent of disease.

Premarin: A brand name for an estrogen medication that is isolated from the urine of pregnant mares. It was introduced in 1941 and was the first estrogen to become widely available to the public.

prosthetic device: Prosthetic devices can be used inside or outside the skin. Tissue expanders and breast implants are placed under the skin to re-create a breast. External prostheses are also available to patients. These are placed inside a bra to create the appearance of a breast.

punch biopsy: A technique used to take a full-thickness sample of skin. A circular cutting blade is attached to a pencil-like handle. The instrument is rotated through the skin and a small disc of tissue is removed. A single suture is often needed to close the incision.

R

radiation: There are four types:

1. **External beam radiation:** The most common type of radiation and the one that has been used for decades. A high-energy beam is directed to the entire breast. The beams are directed at two different angles to avoid damage to the lung and heart. Treatments are daily Monday through Friday and last for six to seven weeks.
2. **Boost dose radiation:** An extra dose of radiation that is given to the area where the cancer was originally located. It can be effective in lowering rates of local recurrence.
3. **Partial breast irradiation:** This form of radiation is directed to the area of the breast where the cancer was originally located. It is typically done a week or more after the surgery and involves inserting a radioactive "seed" into the breast twice a day for five days.
4. **Intraoperative radiation (IORT):** The radiation "seed" is placed into the operative cavity and the radiation is given at the time of the surgical removal of the breast cancer.

randomized clinical trial (RCT): A type of scientific experiment in which the people being studied are randomly allocated to one or another of the different treatments under study (e.g., mammogram versus no mammogram). The RCT is often considered the gold standard for a clinical trial.

S

saline implants: A type of breast implant filled with the same saltwater solution that a patient receives through an IV.

scoliosis: Scoliosis is a sideways curvature of the spine that occurs most often during the growth spurt just before puberty. In most cases the cause of scoliosis is unknown.

screening mammogram: X-rays of the breast that are used to detect breast cancers that are so small they cannot be felt by the woman or her doctor.

sentinel node: The sentinel lymph node, located in the axilla, is the first lymph node that breast cancer cells go to when they spread beyond the breast. If the sentinel node is found to be negative, it is assumed that no other lymph nodes are involved and the removal of more lymph nodes is not required.

silent carriers: Individuals who carry a BRCA1/2 mutation and are unaware of any family history of breast or ovarian cancer.

silicone gel implants: A type of breast implant filled with a silicone gel. Silicone implants are more widely used than saline implants and have been proven to be safe for both cosmetic and reconstruction patients.

solid breast lump: A mass made up of tissue rather than fluid, as is the case with a breast cyst. In most cases a core needle biopsy is used to determine whether a solid lump is malignant or benign (non-cancerous).

spontaneous regression: The partial or complete disappearance of a malignant tumor in the absence of all treatment. Spontaneous regression is a rare event. It has been estimated that it occurs in approximately 1 in 100,000 cancers. There is not a single well-documented case of spontaneous regression occurring in women with breast cancer.

sporadic breast cancers: Cancers that occur in women with no family history of breast cancer. Causes of sporadic cancers are for the most part unknown.

steroids: Topical steroid creams are anti-inflammatory medications that are commonly used to treat skin conditions of the nipple. They should only be applied for a limited time period. If inflammation of the nipple persists after ten days of application, a punch biopsy should be performed.

T

tamoxifen: A pill used to prevent breast cancer in high-risk women. It is also commonly used to treat patients who have been diagnosed with breast cancer and have estrogen-positive tumors.

tissue transfer: Involves moving tissue, typically fat or muscle, from one part of the body to another as part of a reconstruction.

tomosynthesis: A digital mammogram that creates a three-dimensional image of the breast. Allows for better visualization of breast tissue and identification of cancers missed on standard 2-D mammograms.

TRAM flap: Like the DIEP flap, this procedure moves belly fat to the chest to reconstruct a breast. This surgery causes some damage to the rectus muscle and can therefore decrease core strength.

trauma: A physical injury such as occurs in an automobile accident, gunshot wound, or fall. Trauma as referred to in this book does not include psychological trauma.

trauma center: A specialized hospital that treats victims of physical trauma, including blunt trauma from automobile accidents and penetrating trauma that occurs with gunshot injuries. It was my experience with multidisciplinary trauma teams that inspired me to start a multidisciplinary breast care center.

trimester: Pregnancy is typically divided into three periods or trimesters. Each lasts approximately three months. The first trimester is the period of rapid organ development. It is the time period when the developing fetus is most susceptible to exposure to environmental toxins.

triple negative breast cancer: A breast cancer that tests negative for estrogen, progesterone, and HER2+.

tummy tuck: Also called abdominoplasty, a procedure that removes the loose skin and fat from the lower part of the belly. During this procedure the "six-pack" muscles that get stretched apart by pregnancy are usually sewn back together to help restore the shape of the abdomen.

tumor aggressiveness: Refers to breast cancers that are fast growing and more likely to spread to other parts of the body if not appropriately treated.

tumor boards: Multidisciplinary conferences including breast imagers, pathologists, surgeons, oncologists, and other members of the treatment team that meet on regular occasions. The goal is to provide breast cancer patients with a comprehensive treatment plan.

Tyrer-Cuzick model: A risk assessment model, also known as IBIS, that takes into account multiple risk factors including a detailed family history, hormonal factors, and previous biopsy results. It has the highest accuracy of all the risk assessment tools.

U

ultrasound: Breast ultrasound is an imaging technique used to screen for tumors and other breast abnormalities. The ultrasound uses high-frequency sound waves to produce live images of the inside of the breast. Diagnostic ultrasound is used to evaluate a specific area of concern in the breast, while screening ultrasound is used to evaluate both breasts in women who have no known breast problems.

V

variant of unknown significance: A gene mutation that is currently not associated with an increased risk of developing breast cancer.

vitamin D: A vitamin that helps the body absorb calcium, which is essential for good bone health. The skin makes most of your body's vitamin D in response to exposure to sunlight. Low vitamin D levels may be associated with an increased risk of developing breast cancer.

W

wire localization: The process of placing a wire into an abnormal area of the breast that is not palpable but requires surgical removal.

X

X-ray: A high-energy wave that can be used to make images of the body. A mammogram uses X-rays to make images of the breast and identify cancers that cannot be detected on clinical examination.

Index

About the Authors

John G. West, MD, is the director of surgery at Breastlink Orange. A general surgeon by training, Dr. West became fascinated with the multidisciplinary team approach to breast cancer care in the mid-1980s. His previous experience as a pioneer in the development of regional trauma systems set the stage for his interest in developing a team approach to breast care.

Dr. West opened Orange County's first breast care center in 1988, and over the past twenty-five years has been on the cutting edge of refining a team approach to the care of patients with breast problems.

Dr. West was born in Texas and raised in San Francisco. He did his undergraduate work at the University of California, Berkeley, and continued medical and surgical training at the University of California, San Francisco, where he graduated in the top 10 percent of his class. He started to practice in Orange County in 1973.

Dr. West has been named a Best Doctor in America and has been recognized as one of the "Best Doctors in Orange County." He has been the lead author in twenty peer-reviewed articles and has written two books.

Dr. West continues to be at the forefront of cutting-edge breast care issues. He was co-founder and chairman of the board of the Be Aware Foundation, a community outreach program dedicated to the early detection of breast cancer. He has recently been inspired by the work of Michael Porter (author of *Redefining Health Care*) and has made a personal commitment to adapting Porter's principles of value-based competition to the breast care marketplace.

Dr. West and his wife, Jan, have two sons—Justin, Breastlink's director of plastic and reconstructive services, and Matthew, an executive in real estate and finance. Dr. West's interests include physical fitness, gardening, and scuba diving. He is a workaholic who often jokes that his favorite saying is, "Thank God it's Monday."

Maralys Wills has lived three distinct lives: author of sixteen published books (fiction and nonfiction), teacher of college students, and mother of six children—five boys and a girl.

Educated at Stanford and UCLA, she is married to a retired trial attorney. She currently teaches novel writing on the college level, and in 2000 was named Teacher of the Year.

Her most challenging project, a poignant memoir titled *Higher than Eagles*, became her biggest triumph, garnering excellent reviews and five movie options—including from Finnegan-Pinchuk (producers of *Northern Exposure*) and Disney. Currently the book is again under consideration for a feature-length movie.

Several of Wills's books have won national awards: *Damn the Rejections*, *Full Speed Ahead: The Bumpy Road to Getting Published* was named Best Book in its Category from Best Books. Readers on Amazon have been generous in their critiques. Other works have been finalists in Reader's Digest competitions.

Wills considers public speaking the dessert for all the hard work of writing. Contact her: maralys@cox.net or www.maralys.com.

breastlink

Breastlink (www.breastlink.com) is a network of comprehensive breast health centers dedicated to providing optimal care for women.

At our breast care centers in Southern California we offer full-service breast cancer treatment, from initial screenings to the successful completion of treatment. When you walk through our doors you can rest assured that you will be treated with the highest quality of care by breast-dedicated professionals. Breastlink's integrated network allows you to be comprehensively treated by our multidisciplinary team of cancer doctors (including breast imagers, breast surgeons, and reconstructive plastic surgeons, as well as medical and radiation oncologists). Our support team includes a psychotherapist, a nutritionist, and comprehensive in-house volunteer support.

Breastlink also sponsors our research foundation, Cancer Research Collaboration (cancerresearchcollaboration.org), and participates in a wide variety of clinical trials.